# Raw Food Formula for Health

## A Modern Approach to Health through Simplicity, Variety, and Moderation

### by Paul Nison

Healthy Living Publications
Summertown, Tennessee

Cover design:      Warren Jefferson
Interior design:  Gwynelle Dismukes
Cover photo: Sam Sheppard

Everybody's Favorite Salad, page 106, Sweet Annie Kale Salad, page 106, Spanish
"Rice," page 110, Chinese Broccoli with Pine Nuts, page 111, and Strawberry
"Cheesecake," page 116, from *How We All Went Raw* by Charles, Coralanne, and
George Nungesser. Recipes used with permission from the authors.

Published by
Healthy Living Publications
P.O. Box 99
Summertown, TN 38483
1-888-260-8458

Printed in Canada
ISBN  978-1-57067-216-3

13  12  11  10  09  08            6 5 4 3 2 1

      Library of Congress Cataloging-in-Publication Data
Nison, Paul.
  Raw food formula for health : a modern approach through simplicity, variety, and
moderation / by Paul Nison.
      p. cm.
  Includes bibliographical references.
  ISBN 978-1-57067-216-3
  1.  Raw food diet.  I. Title.
  RM237.5.N568 2008
  613.2'6--dc22                          2008007479

We are a member of Green Press Initiative.  We chose to print this title on paper with postconsumer
recycled content, processed without chlorine, which saved the following natural resources:

| | |
|---|---|
| 1,365 pounds of solid waste | 10,631 gallons of water |
| 2,561 pounds of greenhouse gases | 29 trees |
| 20 million BTU of energy | |

**green press** INITIATIVE

For more information, visit <www.greenpressinitiative.org>. Savings calculations thanks to the
Environmental Defense Paper Calculator, <www.papercalculator.org>.

This book is dedicated to
The Durian.
You have changed my life
forever!

# Contents

# Foreword

Paul Nison's fresh contribution to those in the search for better health provides down-to-earth, effective, common-sense approaches to well-being. Each word represents the success he attained after conquering a so-called incurable disorder. There is no better person to speak on the issue of health than someone who has achieved it. We are all caught in the ever-increasing challenges caused by high-speed living and thoughtless emotion. Illness pervades our society, touching even the youngest members. The Western world is plagued with cancer, heart disease, diabetes, gastrointestinal distress, and emotional problems. These escalating maladies are just the tip of the iceberg, reflecting the lack of responsibility the average person maintains for his or her health.

One-third of young married couples struggle to conceive children, and this number is increasing as the years pass. School children are administered psychiatric drugs to tame behavior that is a result of the haphazard lifestyles that their parents lead. Hospital systems and medical facilities are stretched beyond their capabilities. It seems that the "powers that be" do not have the insight, resources, or consciousness to demand a critically needed change in our dietary habits, emotional health, and physical fitness. The whole of modern humanity appears to be addicted to a treadmill lifestyle. The relentless and fruitless pursuit of happiness in the wrong places is maiming our very souls.

As Paul points out in *The Formula for Health*, it is up to us to raise ourselves beyond perceived circumstances and embrace a new paradigm of strength, focused determination, and abundant joy. As you'll learn in this important volume, there are no limits other than those you impose upon yourself. Use this book as a guide to a better you, and remember that the advice offered is not theological, but clinically and personally proven by

Paul and the Institute that I have had the privilege to direct for nearly thirty years. Make sure that you develop enough self-respect to take on all that you do with integrity. Becoming the person you dream of will give you the strength to contribute to and help elevate the human condition.

Thank you, Paul, for being a sane voice among the "health" salesmen who are generally only interested in self-reward. Thank you for speaking from the heart and allowing truth to be your message. Most importantly, thank you for sharing with others.

Brian Clement, PhD, LNC
Director, Hippocrates Health Institute

# Acknowledgments

First, a very special thanks to my wife, Andrea—the most beautiful woman in the world—a true blessing to my life.

Special thanks go to:

All my friends, who have been praying for me through the years. Although far too many to name here, I'm so grateful for your help and friendship.

All the health educators I've interviewed or whose books I've read on the raw food diet and/or the field of health improvement.

Health Research Books for their remarkable stock of the best, hard-to-find health books, and for the permission they granted to quote specific passages.

The Nungessers for their support, prayers, and great recipes.

All the authors in my bibliography, whose information has served as a vast reference and inspiration.

My editor, Carol Wiley Lorente, who has put the finishing touches to my writings, fine-tuning them into a well-written book.

Joel Brody, former Italian professor at Cornell University, Ithaca, New York, for having spent much time guiding me toward the niceties of the English language, for working on the original manuscript of this book, and for his valuable research on Luigi Cornaro.

My publisher, Book Publishing Company, for believing in my work.

Dr. Fred Bisci, who has generously shared his wisdom, friendship, and prayers, and who is ever available to give uplifting advice.

Brian Clement and the Hippocrates Health Institute for being there when I needed them.

All the members of my family, who have always been supportive no matter how much they might not have fully agreed with my ideas.

Above all, our Heavenly Father YHWH. Hallelujah!

# Introduction

I have a most exciting life, traveling the world, studying my favorite topic: health. After my own amazing healing experience, I developed a thrilling passion for sharing messages of hope and healing with everyone I meet. I believe my calling in life is to help people realize that avoiding and overcoming disease is not difficult. It can be simple and even fun.

In any given month, I spend many days lecturing, writing, and helping people create successful, individualized plans to overcome their health challenges. My experiences led me to write several books about the wonderful healing powers of the human body. My passion for healthful food led me to fulfill another dream: I became a chef, creating wonderfully tasty dishes using only the highest-quality foods and ingredients. Working as a chef helps me develop practical ways to make healthful foods enjoyable and food preparation easy to understand.

This book can help you discover how to improve your health and live a disease-free life. The more you understand nutrition's role in preventing disease and curing it, the easier it will be for you to eat healthfully, emphasizing vibrant, live foods. This book will:

1. give you sensible health information that can easily be applied to your life right away;

2. supply the resources to support you on your journey and help keep you on track;

3. teach you a simple formula for health, along with a four-step program to enable you to achieve your goals.

In preparation for writing this book, I studied numerous books by health writers from the past to learn about their medical histories in light of their diet and health recommendations. I talked to health seekers from many parts of the world who have maintained a raw food diet for many years, some for more than fifty years. Many of these interesting interviews are contained in my first three books: *The Raw Life: Becoming*

*Natural in an Unnatural World, Raw Knowledge: Enhancing the Power of the Mind, Body and Soul*, and *Raw Knowledge 2: Interviews with Health Achievers*. These nutrition experts have made it a point throughout their lives to stay in touch with their bodies, continually fine-tuning their diets and making the changes necessary to stay healthy. They are all still thriving today. Their research, confirmed by my own, resulted in this book.

But health isn't just about diet. Along with nutrition, becoming more aware of our emotions and spiritual feelings can truly take our health to another level. My personal experiences with nutrition and healing have thrilled me to no end, but it's my personal relationship with Our Creator that has truly blessed me.

I am excited to present this information to you. I know it will help you reach your goals of health and wellness. Here's to your ongoing enjoyment of consistently improving health!

Paul Nison

# Chapter 1

# My Road to Health

I have not always been healthy. I was barely out of my teens when I was diagnosed with a so-called incurable illness. I've seen the inside of more than a few emergency rooms, and I've been shunted from doctor to doctor in a search for answers to my pain and disease. It took a lot of personal medical sleuthing and research before I came upon my own cure for my illness. Since then, I have enjoyed good health and have dedicated my life to helping others have it, too.

As a young man, I had always been fit; a gym rat, I never missed my daily workout. I was trim and buff, muscular and in shape, and always working out, but, as I would discover at the tender age of twenty, I was far from healthy. Suddenly, I began having severe stomach pains and diarrhea. The pain became so bad that I went to the emergency room; the doctors said I had food poisoning and sent me home.

The pain and diarrhea went on for several days—sometimes I couldn't leave the bathroom for hours—and every time I saw a doctor or went to an emergency room, I was diagnosed with food poisoning. (Little did I know how prophetic the words "food poisoning" would be. Yes, I had "food poisoning," but not the way my doctors would have defined it!) Finally, after the most painful bout I had experienced, I was diagnosed with inflammatory bowel disease, an umbrella term that includes ulcerative colitis and Crohn's disease. I was told there was no known medical cure for either of these conditions, and I was given some medication that I was told I'd have to take for the rest of my life.

Inflammatory bowel disease (IBD) entails a combination of intermittent abdominal pain, constipation, and diarrhea, and results in structural changes to the intestines. Ulcerative colitis is a chronic inflammation and ulceration of the colon lining. In Crohn's disease, the colon lining thickens due to prolonged inflammation; it is believed to be an autoimmune disease. Most medical doctors do not know what causes these diseases, nor can they cure them; mostly, they are managed with drugs and, in severe cases, surgery to remove parts of the intestines.

I began taking the medications, but the side effects were so uncomfortable that I again sought help from doctors, who gave me more medications to counter the side effects. Before I knew it, I was taking more drugs than my grandmother. I also noticed something very interesting: I kept running into the same group of people in doctors' waiting rooms. It seemed like we were all members of a little club that went from specialist to specialist in a vain search for relief. Our diseases weren't being cured; they were only being managed.

## Overnight Vegan

Growing up, I ate the standard American diet. Mostly, I lived on pizza; sometimes I ate pizza three times a day. I had no idea that what I was eating had anything to do with my illness, but after I was diagnosed, people began to ask me if what I ate affected my condition in any way. Increasingly, it seemed logical that what I ate would have some effect on my illness, but my doctors repeatedly told me there were no studies to indicate that what I ate would make any difference.

I tried everything to get rid of my illness, because I realized that I had to change what I was doing to change the results. Someone told me that dairy products were the worst offenders. Dairy products made up about 80 percent of my diet, and my doctor said there was no medical evidence that dairy products caused these problems. Without telling my doctor, I decided to eliminate dairy products from my diet. I started getting better.

Then I heard that meat could be causing my problems, so I asked the doctor if becoming a vegetarian would help me. She said there were no medical studies that indicated that eliminating meat would improve anything. I became a vegan literally overnight; but, because I didn't yet understand much about nutrition, I was a junk food vegan. Even so, I began to feel better.

It seemed that every time the doctor told me something, I'd do the opposite and get better. So, when she told me there were no medical studies that indicated that stress contributed to my problems, I "eliminated" my doctor to reduce the ongoing stress in my life. I quit my job and moved from my high-stress hometown of Brooklyn, New York, to the least stressful place I could find, West Palm Beach, Florida.

After a couple of weeks in Florida, I began to notice a van in my neighborhood with "Hippocrates" painted on the side. I was so intrigued that, one day, I followed it to see where it was going. The van pulled up outside a natural food store and several people got out. They were going inside for a tour and I decided to tag along. What I learned that day would change my life.

## My First Inspiration

The Hippocrates Health Institute was founded in 1956 by Ann Wigmore, a visionary and humanitarian who became the world's leading authority on the raw and live food diet. She established Hippocrates as a place where people could spend one to three weeks immersed in a lifestyle that emphasizes raw food, positive thinking, and noninvasive therapies on the path to optimum health. Hippocrates' goal is to help us realize that good health is every person's birthright, that we are all entitled to a life free of disease and pain.

But as I accompanied the vanload of tourists into the health food store that day, I wasn't sure that their program was something I could ever do. That's because Brian Clement, the Hippocrates director, who was leading the tour, immediately shepherded all of us over to the produce section and started telling us how important it is that most of our diet consist of these things. But I hated fruits and vegetables. Yes, I was a vegan, but I was a junk food vegan: I ate a lot of highly processed soy foods and organic cookies and smoothies and such, but I didn't eat fruits or vegetables. So I asked him, "What happens if you don't like fruits and vegetables?" He told me that, since I lived in the neighborhood, I should come to Hippocrates for a visit.

As I entered the Hippocrates Institute on the day of my visit, I saw a woman in a wheelchair. She looked very ill, and I worried that perhaps Brian Clement wasn't telling me the whole story about this place. If such a sick person as this isn't getting better, maybe the program is not what it was cracked up to be. Nevertheless, wanting to keep an open mind, and still searching for a cure for my own illness, I went home with an armload of their books and videos. As a result of what I read in the books and saw in the videos, I decided to begin their three-week program. As I arrived at the center, I noticed a woman jogging on the grounds. To my amazement, it was the woman I had seen in the wheelchair just weeks earlier. At that moment, I had the tremendously exciting feeling that I knew I was going to get well.

## Raw, Ripe, Fresh, and Organic

Before I got sick, I ate a lot of harmful food, but I felt fine, so I didn't care. When I got sick and took steps to get well by eliminating animal products from my diet, I realized health doesn't start with what we *add* to our diet—it starts with what we leave *out*. There is a prevalent mistaken belief these days that, to achieve good health, it's important to add foods, drinks, medicines, and/or supplements to what we're already consuming. Although some of these things can be helpful in certain situations, the key to health is not adding more to your current diet but leaving out the harmful, problem-causing stuff. As I eliminated more and more unhealthful foods, the healthful foods I was left with were raw, ripe, fresh, and organic fruits, vegetables, nuts, and seeds.

As a result of what I learned at Hippocrates, my "incurable" disease was cured. I was amazed at how quickly my health returned, particularly because my doctor had warned me that a diet of raw fruits and vegetables would be harmful to anyone with inflammatory bowel disease. (Doctors still tell IBD patients not to eat acidic fruits and some raw vegetables, particularly lettuce and other leafy greens.) Yet I learned that simple fruits and vegetables of the highest quality were all I needed to be healthy. That's why I like to call my diet a "high-quality diet" rather than a "raw food diet," because the highest-quality food we can consume is food that has not been cooked.

Over the years, this diet has kept my disease away and left me feeling healthy and energetic. We will discuss this in greater depth in chapter 4, but, put quite simply, the elements of this diet are these:

- **Eat raw food.** Why? Raw, uncooked food is also called "live" (rhymes with "thrive") food because it contains active enzymes. I think of enzymes as the energy and life of the food. Enzymes are keys that unlock the door to your body's energy supplies: Without enzymes, your body uses more energy than it should to get vital nutrients from the food you eat. Cooking food not only kills the enzymes, it also causes the water in the food to evaporate. The more cooked food we eat, the more water we need to drink.
- **Eat fresh foods**. As soon as a fruit or vegetable is picked, it begins losing nutrients and enzymes, so food should be eaten as close to the time

of picking as possible. In today's world, unless you grow the food yourself, this can be tricky. But with all the emphasis these days on "eating locally," it is getting easier to find really fresh foods, at least during the warmer months. Farmers markets are great places for buying truly fresh produce, because the growers usually pick the vegetables and fruits they sell only hours before they bring it to market. Find out where your food comes from. For example, if you live in the Midwest and the produce at your supermarket comes from Chile, you might want to shop around for a source that's closer to home.

- **Eat ripe food**. Another reason you want to select produce grown closer to home is because when food has to travel hundreds or thousands of miles to get to your supermarket from the field, it is picked before it's ripe so it can ripen—but not overripen—on the way to market. But picking produce before its time doesn't give it a chance to ripen the way it would if it were left on the vine or branch. Nutritionally, there's a big difference between tree- and vine-ripened fruits and vegetables and those that are picked prematurely. A fruit will naturally fall from the tree when it is ready to fall, and at that point, it is packed with nutrients and enzymes. It also tastes much better. A big reason why I never liked fruits and vegetables in the past was because my supermarkets didn't carry produce that was naturally ripe.

- **Eat organic food**. There are more reasons to eat organic food than just to avoid synthetic fertilizers and pesticides. Although these reasons are important—you certainly can't be healthy if you're ingesting pesticide residues—agricultural chemicals contaminate the soil and destroy natural nutrients found in it. As a result, plants grown in chemically depleted soil will be less nutritious than organic food grown in nutrient-rich soil.

It's important to remember that it's not just the type of food consumed but also the amount and quality that counts. My Formula for Health prescribes a diet of the highest-quality foods—consumed in their simplest forms—that enable the human body to function in utmost harmony with its design. Think of it this way: When you put cheap gas in your car, it doesn't run very well; it just kind of chugs along. The cheap fuel doesn't keep your engine clean, and your car might not get the best gas mileage. Treat your body like you would an expensive automobile. High-quality fuel in the form of raw, ripe, fresh, organic fruits, vegetables, nuts, and seeds will keep your "engine" running smoothly for longer periods, and, as we'll discuss in chapter 3, it will keep your body "cleaner" as well.

## SO MANY DIETS

One of the stresses of modern life is what I call the "paradox of choice." It seems like every time we decide we want to do something, we are faced with so many choices that we're just not sure which one is right for us. Ideally, we should study every choice and then use the wisdom we would gain to make a decision. But there are usually so many choices that sometimes it just isn't feasible or practical to do the research we'd need to figure it out.

A diet plan for health is no different. Today, there are many different popular diets—the Blood Type Diet, the Atkins Diet, the Beverly Hills Diet—all with success stories. If all of them work, how do we know which one to follow? The fact is, any diet can deliver results to a degree because they all eliminate some harmful foods. The reason you should choose the Formula for Health is because it eliminates *all* harmful foods. Following the formula for health explained in this book is a safe and quick way to get well and stay well.

## Feed the Spirit, Too

No matter how good your diet is, there is more to being healthy than the food you eat. You should not make food the focus of your health program to the exclusion of everything else. You cannot be completely healthy without taking care of the emotional and spiritual aspects of your life. I didn't know it at the time, but my return to health and a simpler life was just the beginning of a path that would bring me to question the connection between today's fast-paced urban lifestyle and the sad, diseased state in which so many people find themselves. The more I started to realize what was really going on, the more I saw most people moving around like robots, barely surviving while I was thriving. I had a new understanding of "less is more."

My search for a better life also led me on a spiritual path that put me on a mission to bring the message of health and healing to everyone. I began writing books about health, traveling around the world, lecturing about health and living simply, and assuring people that they can have a healing like I have had. I read the Scriptures, began a personal relationship with Our Creator, and discovered that the Bible is the greatest book on health ever written.

The investment you make in your health can create a wonderful life of happiness and wellness. The Formula for Health can give you that life by providing the program you need. As a fitness specialist, I have to follow a well-balanced program. If I didn't, I wouldn't have a balanced body; my chest and arms might be fit and muscular, while my legs might be poorly developed and weak. You need to do the same—develop a balanced program based on the Formula for Health and make a decision to follow it. It's easy to be disciplined about something we love, something we're passionate about. We need to find that passion for good health.

Following a healthful diet requires a little more knowledge than just eating raw fruits and vegetables (we'll get into that in greater depth in chapter 3). But before we talk about getting healthy, we need to understand how we get sick in the first place.

# Chapter 2

# What is Disease?

*The Human Body is governed by Natural Law. We have to live within Natural Law. It's the same thing as if you tried to jump out of a plane without a parachute; there's a law of aerodynamics and gravity, and there's the wind factor. And, if you jump out, despite thinking you're a canary, you're going to hit the ground.*

*—Fred Bisci, Ph.D., clinical nutritionist*
*and raw foodist for over fifty years*

I lecture about health and wellness all over the world. When I give my lectures, I find that most people are concerned with three things:

1. How to cure disease

2. How to prevent disease

3. How to stay young looking

People are always surprised—and relieved—to know that the cure for their illness is within their grasp and absolutely under their control. The human body is the most intelligently designed machine out there, and, like any machine, if we take care of it, it will last a very long time and serve us well. If we neglect it, however, it will break down. Fortunately, like most machines, the body can be repaired, and, most of the time it will return to a smooth-running state. Then, if we just listen to our bodies and respond correctly, we can expect to be healthy—and young looking—for a very long time.

Disease is a great warning sign that alerts us to what is happening inside our bodies. How reassuring it is to know that, if we catch it early enough, we are in full control of the cure. I've seen hundreds of people make healing a passion; I've experienced it myself. And I have known people with the most serious of illnesses who have fully recovered once they've applied a wise approach to their healing program. With a few simple steps, you can too. Don't always rely on the drug-centered medical system to "cure" you; most of the time, drugs merely treat the symptoms, not the disease. You deserve—and can attain—better than that.

We need to try to get at the root cause of disease. If you can understand what is causing your illness, you stand a better chance of overcoming it. Once you do overcome it, you'll be able to avoid any future issues with your health, and looking young and staying healthy will most likely come naturally.

## Why We Get Sick

People may not like to hear it, but most disease is self-inflicted. We get sick anytime we violate natural law—the biological laws governing the human body and the laws of a sound mind—or, I believe, when we go against Scriptural laws. Violations of these laws, even to a minor degree, will result in impaired health. Looked at another way, though, this works in our favor; it means we can cure ourselves.

Learning about the design of the body and how it is supposed to work is the best foundation for developing a health plan. Then you can take the first step: determining the root cause of your health problem. I believe the following three areas are the root causes of disease:

- Spiritual: a lack of faith and understanding of the Divine
- Emotional: mental stress, anxiety, and the paradox of choice
- Physical: overeating, poor diet, and lack of sufficient exercise, water, and sound sleep

Most people know when something is wrong because they feel pain. Obviously, if you drop a hammer on your foot, you will resolve to be more careful in the future; there isn't much reason to revamp your entire lifestyle to handle that sort of injury. But I don't necessarily mean "pain" in the classic sense of a sharp or chronic stabbing sensation, but rather a feeling of discomfort that indicates there is something that's just not right. I prefer to call this "pain" because, frankly, it's not "disease" people want to avoid per se; it's the pain and discomforts that come with disease that make them want to find a cure.

People who understands how the human body works are better able to figure out what it is they're doing wrong and take action to stop the cause. Usually, stopping the cause alone will start the healing; other times, the body may also need rest to heal. There are occasions when additional interventions may be needed.

But sometimes illness can be quite subtle. Years of living on an inadequate or harmful diet can cause a delayed reaction, damaging our health but perhaps not producing "pain" until disease has advanced to a point where we're really seriously ill. In these cases, many people lose the great blessing of health before they even realize what's happened.

People will seek help right away if they're in an accident or if they're suddenly in great pain, but in the case of seemingly minor discomfort or a subtle illness, people usually wait until the pain is so bad they cannot bear it. Then they may run to the doctor, who may attempt to control the illness with drugs. The problem is that, most of the time, drugs will only temporarily suppress symptoms, and this is not a cure. The discomfort might be controlled for a while, but it could come back even worse. The wise person will figure out what the cause is and deal with it immediately.

Most people today experience many discomforts from eating a low-quality diet, yet they ignore the pleadings of their body to eat better. Instead, they continue to stuff themselves until the body adapts to the poor diet and they've lost their ability to feel the warning signs. This, coupled with the fact that almost everyone else around them is eating the same way, results in a fantasy that nothing is wrong. The patient continues to exacerbate the condition until he or she ends up in the advanced stages of discomfort or disease, only to wonder how this could have happened.

## The Power of Adaptation

*The body's ability to adapt is remarkable, but health is a delusion when you attempt to produce it by drugs. Under such circumstances, the body will inevitably become exhausted and chronic illness will ensue.*

—*Fred Bisci, Ph.D.*

How wonderful to know that we can be cured of many diseases simply by avoiding harmful foods. And what's even more fascinating is how we can eat harmful foods for years and not get sick. The body is amazing and has astounding power to adapt to any situation.

Adaptation is a wonderful survival tool if it is used properly; but if we use it incorrectly, we can receive the false impression that everything is fine, even when it may not be. The body is so perfectly equipped with the power of adaptation that it will adjust itself, in time, to tolerate harmful food and a toxic environment. Health author Hilton Hotema offers this pertinent example: Most people today live in environments with poor-quality air, but the majority of us breathe without noticeable discomfort because our lungs have adapted to it. If people with healthy lungs, such as very young children, were forced to breathe in the same unhealthful air, their bodies might find it unbearable. Because of the body's power of adaptation, people can live in polluted air and, on the surface, appear to suffer nothing more than coughs, colds, hay fever, sore throats, and other relatively mild ailments of the respiratory organs. Yet, they may be slowly dying from the effects of that air and don't realize it; they have become "immune." Immunity is the ability to adapt to a condition or tolerate a poison that doesn't kill us on the spot.

Just as the body has an amazing power to adapt to its environment, it also has an amazing power to adapt to a poor diet. The more your body adapts—that is, the more that toxins build up in your body—the less sensitive, or less responsive, it will be to harmful living and the less capable it will be of producing warning signs that you are diseased; it will only be capable of producing weaker warning signs. But the cleaner (that is, the fewer toxins your body contains) and healthier your body becomes, the better it will react should you encounter something harmful. This is the state we all want to achieve, and with the Formula for Health, we can reach that goal.

We've all heard someone who eats a very poor diet say that he never gets sick. It may very well be true, at least for now, because his body has adapted. It's not that he is just one of the "lucky ones," however. One day his bad eating habits will catch up to him, because adaptation can occur only at the expense of the body's vital functions; it has to change the body in a negative way in order to reach immunity. And if the body continues to adapt to poisons and harmful food, the adaptation itself becomes toxic to us as well. Hotema tells us, "It's in this condition that people slowly get sicker and sicker while being treated for some 'disease.' There is no mystery to this: if you keep doing the same thing, you will keep getting the same result, and the damage will just go deeper and deeper." We have to learn how to change our actions and limit the poisons we ingest so we can get and remain healthy.

Most people today are so internally "dirty" that they've lost the ability to feel pain and sense disease. For example, overeating poor-quality food for years will result in a buildup of mucus and toxins in our tissues. I contend that this excess amount of internal waste is a common cause of disease. The body does its best to rid itself of these toxins if we let it do its job. Instead, many people suppress the toxic waste from being released; case in point is the example of the common cold. People take antihistamines to dry up their runny noses, cough medicine to suppress their coughs, and pain relievers to ease their aches and pains. Instead of understanding that the body is trying to eliminate toxins, they are led to believe they are sick. In actuality, they are creating a more toxic environment and making the illness worse.

Every sneeze, every cough, every cold, and every headache are the first warning signs that you are diseased. The next common signals are exhaustion and constipation. Listening to the body is a safe way to tell if we are doing something wrong, but it will only respond correctly when it has been detoxified, or internally cleaned. Later in this book we will discuss how you can get rid of these toxins through a process called *detoxification*.

## Better To Respond Than Adapt

I have found that the body can adapt to any harmful situation and deal with it, but only for a short while. If we take care of ourselves by not putting harmful substances into our bodies, they will work according to design, always giving us true signs of what's happening internally. Then we can *respond* instead of *adapt*. A healthy body will react to toxic substances, such as junk food, and begin to show signs of pain so that we can respond appropriately and begin to take care of ourselves. We must learn what pain is and understand why we experience discomfort.

Here's an example: If you live on pizza, soda pop, and hot dogs, and your stomach gets upset, you should rest and not put anything else into your system until you feel better. Just as you try to keep the outside of your body from getting dirty, it's equally as important to keep the inside of your body clean. Most of us haven't learned this lesson until we've already developed a "dirty interior." The body will cleanse itself, however, when it is given sufficient time for healing and the proper diet to clear away toxins.

Because our bodies have this amazing ability to adapt—to continue feeling good and looking great even while a health issue is brewing—we may need a blood test to uncover specific problems, especially more subtle ones. The blood is a great messenger and can reveal what is taking place deep inside the body. If a nutritional deficiency is brought to light, we can obtain the missing nutrients through our diets and address any resultant damage. If the problem persists, we then need to look at emotional issues as a possible cause. Don't hesitate to seek counseling if you have a problem that may be related to stress, depression, or anxiety that you can't get a handle on by yourself. Finally, if the problem is not the result of physical or emotional issues, there may be a spiritual concern that needs to be dealt with. Perhaps all three areas—physical, emotional, and spiritual—will need your attention.

Sometimes it seems as though new diseases are popping up every day. Have you ever wondered how there could be so many different diseases when most people are disobeying the same laws of health? It has always been my contention that there is only one disease with many different stages. I have come to the conclusion that, beginning with fatigue and ending in cancer, the "different diseases" are simply different levels, or progressions, of the same disease.

The good news is that, in many cases, the damage can be reversed, as long as we start to pay attention to the laws of health. No one should ever give up, no matter how serious the disease may be, because as long as the body still has the vital energy to heal itself, there is hope. (More about this in chapter 3.)

Most diseases, in my opinion, have clear warning signals and progress in distinct stages. We just need to heed these stages early on and realize they are truly serious; then we can deal with them wisely so the problem doesn't move to the next level. Natural hygiene doctors have identified the following as the stages of cancer. But I believe there is only one disease—beginning with exhaustion and ending in cancer—so I have adapted these stages as the progression of *all* disease:

1. Exhaustion
2. Toxemia (in the form of constipation)
3. Irritation
4. Inflammation
5. Ulceration
6. Induration (in the form of a hardened mass)
7. Fungation (in the form of cancer)

## Exhaustion and Constipation

I believe the first signs of disease are chronic exhaustion and constipation, so let's consider these together, because usually where there's one, there is also the other.

These first two stages of disease are so common that most people accept them as "normal." But don't become acquiescent about them. The more frequently you experience these stages, the more "normal" you will think they are, and the more difficult it will be to heal from them.

There is a difference between feeling exhausted and being tired. If you work hard and you're tired at the end of the day, that's normal. However, if you're not using much energy during the day and you still feel tired, that's exhaustion. When you wake up, you should be energized and feel excited about life. If you don't, chances are it's because disease is building in your body.

If you feel exhausted and fatigued all the time, if you never feel like doing anything, your energy, and the energy your body needs to operate efficiently, is being depleted. As a result, nerve energy can no longer freely move through the body, resulting in a condition I call "nervous exhaustion." When this happens, toxins get deposited in the body.

There's no secret as to why we might be tired all the time: It is caused by overeating, stress, and a lack of water, proper nutrition, and sleep.

Most fatigued people are constipated, although typically they will deny it. I don't listen to them, because I don't listen to anyone who is full of something, if you get my drift. In fact, I actually met someone who was so tired and exhausted, he was completely content to be constipated because he didn't have to get up and go to the bathroom. I wish I was just joking about that, but it's actually true.

Surprisingly, that person is not alone in his thinking. Many people in the civilized world are constipated, walking around with five to ten pounds of fecal waste in their intestines. The average person has a bowel movement once every other day and thinks that's normal, but just because it's normal for him doesn't mean it's healthy or optimal. I know someone who has only two bowel movements a week and considers that healthy because it's normal for him. Unfortunately, even children in the United States are now becoming exhausted and constipated.

When you are constipated, or not having enough bowel movements each day, toxins begin to accumulate in the blood, tissues, lymphatic system, interstitial fluids, and cells. These toxins impair the functions of your organs and tissues. This state is referred to as *toxemia*, and it is caused by a combination of fatigue, overeating—especially overeating the wrong types of foods—and negative thoughts. The cure is to clean up your diet and clear up your mind. Don't let negativity take control.

Fatigue and constipation indicate the start of more serious conditions, and they shouldn't be ignored or brushed off as minor inconveniences. They have to be cured if we want to overcome or avoid the more advanced and increasingly severe stages of disease.

# Irritation

If you continue to overindulge and ignore your body's messages, toxins will seek out places to hide in your body. They gravitate to places that are already irritated. You'll know when toxins have accumulated to dangerous levels because you may feel itchy, sneezy, queasy, jumpy, or antsy, or you may have intense bodily urges or feelings of arousal, or you may just have a general feeling of annoyance.

Toxic overloads also can also affect your emotional state. You may feel irritable and on edge. This is your body telling you that toxins have accumulated to the point of causing symptoms. Unless you start taking care of yourself—by eating high-quality foods, getting enough rest, and cleansing internally—your body will advance to the next stage of disease. Listen to your body. Be sensible in your diet and lifestyle.

# Inflammation

When an irritation caused by toxemia or injury is not treated, it becomes inflamed. At this stage, you will have noticeable pain and discomfort, and it's usually at this stage that we call a physician. A doctor will often administer drugs to relieve your pain and inflammation, but drugs may only add to the toxic buildup that's continuing in the body. When you feel pain or disease, rest. Relax, sleep, fast, and meditate—that's when the most natural healing takes place.

# Ulceration

An ulcer is characterized by a break in the skin or in a mucous membrane, often accompanied by an accumulation of pus. Canker sores, open sores, and stomach ulcers are common examples. Often, nerves are not only irritated, they may also be exposed, so this condition can be very painful and aggravating. An excessive buildup of toxins necessitates extreme measures to remove them, and I believe the body actually creates these conditions in order to relieve itself of an overabundance of toxic material. At this stage, medical doctors will prescribe potent drugs, and perhaps even perform surgery. But, if the body is permitted to rest, it could still repair the wound naturally and heal itself.

This is a very serious stage in disease progression, because if measures are not taken to detoxify, or cleanse, the body, it may no longer be able to heal itself. At this point, the body can heal only if it has some vital energy left and we give it what it needs: rest, high-quality food, and prayer.

## Indurations

An induration is a hardening. In an attempt to isolate toxins, body tissue will actually harden around them and create sacs, or what are also commonly referred to as polyps, tumors, cysts, and warts. This is the body's defensive move to prevent toxins from contaminating the rest of the body.

At this stage, physical pain and emotional distress intensify. This is the last intelligent activity the body will perform before the final stage of disease—cancer. If not taken care of, the result could be an irreversible form of disease that not even your body can overcome, no matter what natural methods you use. If you don't wake up now, your body may never be able to wake up again.

## Fungation

Cancer is an overgrowth of cells due to a disruption of their genetic encoding by poisonous substances. (It is called "fungation" because the growth and invasion of cancer cells can resemble fungus.) These mutated cells obtain their nourishment from lymph fluid. As long as nourishment is available, cancer cells continue to thrive and divide. This stage is chronic and often irreversible, as the body degenerates past the point of no return.

Regardless of the stage of disease, the cause is always the same: a continuous, long-term saturation of poisons, which compromise cellular integrity. The result is the final phase of disease, which the body can no longer overcome. At this point it is fatal.

Whatever stage of disease your body may be in, never stop trying to heal and eliminate toxins. Give your body the rest it needs. There is no way to tell when it has reached the point of no return, so giving up is never an option. The present moment may be your only chance to help yourself recover.

The good news is, in many cases, the damage can be reversed, as long as we start to pay attention to the laws of health. I think even cancer can be overcome if the body still has enough vital energy to heal. Understanding the Formula for Health and the causes of disease can help our bodies hang on to the vital energy that overcomes illness.

# Chapter 3

# The Formula for Health

*To be truly healthy involves a comprehensive change in one's lifestyle.*
*Everything changes. The body is always changing. It keeps moving. It's*
*either moving backward or forward. If you stop, you are moving back-*
*ward. The human body is always pushing toward perfection. We have the*
*ability to live a life that is so glorious, so far beyond what people could*
*realize. But we must realize that no two people are the same. There are*
*1,000 variables on a daily basis that happen to our body. Two people can*
*be doing the exact same thing and get a different result because of all the*
*different variables out there.*
—*Fred Bisci, Ph.D.*

In 1866, Arnold Ehret was born in Baden, Germany. The son of a gifted
and creative farmer, Ehret also inherited gifts—for chemistry, physics,
drawing, painting, and languages. At age twenty-one, he became a professor of art, a career that was cut short by the military draft. But he was-
n't in the military long, once it was discovered he had heart disease.
Then, at age thirty-one, he was diagnosed with Bright's disease, an
inflammation of the kidneys. He was examined by doctors all over
Europe; each one diagnosed his disease as incurable.

Ehret turned to alternative medicine for help. He visited health sani-
tariums throughout Europe and Africa in a quest to learn about holistic
healing. He discovered that simply eating less made him feel better. It
also gave him greater strength and vitality. Eventually, he credited his
fruit diet and fasting for healing both his heart condition and his kidney
disease.

Ehret opened a sanitarium in Switzerland and became widely known for curing thousands of people whose diseases had been labeled incurable by physicians. He was known for his long periods of fasting, which lasted from three to seven weeks, and for his fruitarian diet. He became one of the most popular health lecturers in Europe, and, in 1914, he brought his knowledge to the United States, where he also lectured and wrote his seminal treatise on diet and health, *The Mucusless Diet Healing System*. ("Mucus" was Ehret's term for toxins; we will use the same definition in this book.) He died at age fifty-six after a fatal head injury resulting from a fall.

Ehret's book is still an inspiration to people who are passionate about health. His diet is expertly planned to transition the patient from a toxic diet to a combination of fasting and healthful, high-quality food. His formula for life provides a brilliantly simple equation that easily sums up how good health is created:

## Vitality = Power - Obstruction

Here's how Ehret's formula works. Health is power, or as I prefer to refer to it, energy. I don't mean energy as in stimulation, but rather the energy you get when you've had the proper sleep and nutrition. Obstruction is disease, and vitality is wellness, or the level of health we experience. So another way to write the formula is:

## Health - Disease = Wellness

In other words, your degree of wellness or vitality is what's left of your health when you "subtract" any sickness or discomfort. For example, if you're a very healthy person and you happen to get a cold, you still have a good supply of overall wellness. But if you don't eat right and you're not sleeping enough, and then you get a cold, you'll have less vitality and a reduced ability to heal. Obviously, the healthier you are, the more vitality you will have to help you when you get sick.

As long as the body is able to maintain enough power/health to remove the obstruction/disease, there is going to be some degree of vitality/wellness. If the obstruction/disease becomes greater than your power/health, you won't have the energy to get rid of the obstruction. The greater the obstruction, the more likely the disease will reach an advanced stage. Thus the state of our health is determined by the degree of this vital energy we have left after the body has used its power to get rid of the waste. If the body runs out of energy to supply the power, waste will build up more quickly. At that point, the body no longer has enough power to eliminate the buildup of toxic substances, and this results in an excess amount of toxins accumulating in the blood. Soon, the first stages of disease are experienced.

If Power - Obstruction = Vitality, too little power and too much obstruction will put us in a very diseased state. This is the essence of the Formula for Health, and, as we'll see, it can help you understand how a high-quality raw food diet, sufficient sleep, and detoxification can keep the obstructions in check and your vitality soaring.

## The Source of Power

Power comes from all the gifts our Creator has given us, which so many of us take for granted. These gifts make our bodies wonderfully strong and amazing machines. The air we breathe, the water we drink, fresh, high-quality food, and sunlight are just some of the many gifts we receive every day. Proper use of these gifts can make us stronger, increasing our power and vitality.

Many daily pressures we experience—poor diet, environmental toxins, emotional stress, and even spiritual confusion and doubt—consume our energy and sap the body's power supply. Unfortunately, there's no reasonable test to conclude how much energy we have or don't have. Science can determine how much vitality we have only to a degree, based on our organ functions and stress levels, but since there are many other factors that indicate vitality, or lack of it, science cannot provide reliable measurements. The good news is that the body stores energy, and very few people will ever reach total energy deprivation as long as they follow nature's laws.

One way to maintain your energy is to allow your body to heal itself without interference. If you impede your body's natural healing mechanisms, it will be forced to expend energy to deal with the interference. As you will begin to understand, the key to conserving energy is to rid yourself of obstructions through fasting (which we will discuss in chapter 5), eating right, and getting enough rest.

A common misconception is that energy, or vitality, means *stimulation*. But stimulation is not vitality. Rather, it is a false source of energy with levels that go up and down depending on what we eat or don't eat. Real energy is always there for us to tap into, unless we do something to use it up. Health, or energy, is not achieved by what we add but by what we get rid of. Health cannot be obtained by eating more highly stimulating foods but by eating fewer of them.

High-quality nutrition, along with maintaining a clean internal environment, will help create and conserve energy/vitality. The key to health from a physical standpoint is taking in as many nutrients as possible while using as little energy as possible to digest them, and also keeping the body's internal environment as clean as possible. Raw fruits and vegetables do just that.

A consistent flow of energy in our body will keep us healthy, vibrant, and excited about life. The more energy we have, the more power we can produce. The first sign of energy drain is the first sign of disease. Let's go back to the car example: no matter how powerful the engine in the car, without gasoline, the car will not go anywhere.

Fruits and vegetables require the least amount of the body's energy to digest, yet they provide the most nutrients. In other words, you get more bang for your buck with fruits and vegetables than with any other foods, and they are your best source of energy conservation.

## Overeating Saps Energy

If we know that obstruction causes a depletion of body energy, what can we do to prevent it? The most common cause for obstruction is overeating: eating too much food and eating too often. In my opinion, this is the leading cause of disease. The second cause is lack of sleep. Too much food in our system cuts into our power base by forcing our body to use energy to store or expel the excess food. Lack of sleep, or "undersleeping," as I like to call it, does not give the body enough time to recharge, also causing a lack of power. Not enough power and too much obstruction put us right into a state of disease.

## How Much To Eat?

Diet books typically pay too much attention to calories while neglecting the importance of high-quality food. A person who eats 3,500 calories' worth of low-quality foods per day can starve for lack of nutrients, but a person who eats higher-quality foods may be well nourished by eating only half that number of calories. The average person engaged in ordinary business and light exercise can maintain health and efficiency very well on a high-quality diet of 2,000 calories per day.

Obviously, the number of calories and nutrients each person requires will vary depending on age, gender, and activity level, but more significant is what foods are needed based on how clean the body is. Someone whose body is full of toxins may need more raw, ripe, fresh, organic food—not for its nutrient content, but to limit the high amount of toxic waste that will be released from the body once a cleansing diet has been initiated. The cleaner a person is or becomes internally, the less waste will be created, and the less food will be required. I've spent time with people who have been eating a very high-quality diet for many years, and they eat very little. They're very active and strong and their minds are sharp. Over the years, I, too, have cut down on the amount of food I consume.

Active people may need more food, but there is no reason for excessive exercise. Too much of a good thing can be harmful. I know people who exercise way too much just so they can eat more. But excess leads to energy loss. Physical exercise is very important on a daily basis, but a person who is eating a high-quality diet and following the formula for health doesn't need to spend as much time and energy exercising as a person who overeats and lives an unhealthful lifestyle.

I believe that once our body is healthy and cleansed, we need very little food, as long as it is good-quality food. Eating two meals a day of raw, ripe, fresh, and organic food, plus two juices made with chlorophyll-rich vegetables, is ideal. This gives the body enough time to properly and fully digest the food. As long as a good variety of food is consumed, and it contains the high-quality nutrients the body needs, there is no need for more.

## The Dangers of Overeating

*Man lives on one-third of what he eats. The doctor lives on the other two-thirds.* —*Anonymous*

Eating for pleasure has replaced the concept of eating for nourishment, and this has led to a society that consumes more food than necessary. The common sign of this is being overweight; an even more common result of overeating is lack of energy.

No activity takes more energy from the body than dealing with too much food. Overeating often causes more obstruction than nutritional intake. It drains our energy, creates disease, and brings toxic-waste gases—a result of the waste trapped in our intestines—into our blood-stream, leading to many deadly problems.

It's not the amount of food that keeps you alive but how much of what you eat that the body actually uses that's important. Excess will cause trouble. You can eat a lot of food and still starve if your cells can't use any of it.

It's very sad that Americans are so conditioned to overconsume food. More money is spent on food each year than on gasoline and medical care combined. Most people could reduce their food intake by half and be healthier. The cleaner the body, the more efficiently it will be able to extract nutrients. The longer you eat raw, ripe, fresh, organic food, the greater your ability to thrive on significantly less food.

> The time of day we consume our meals is also important. If we have an ideal sleeping pattern for health, we will be rising just before sunrise and going to sleep well before the midnight hour (around nine o'clock), so the ideal times to eat our meals would be nine in the morning and three in the afternoon. This might seem odd at first, but give it a try and see how much better you feel. (See chapter 7 for a suggested daily schedule.)

## Why Do People Eat So Much?

*Emaciation is nearly always due to the wasting from disease, not to lack of food. A person who is really ill can continue to waste away, no matter how much food he eats; indeed, he often wastes more rapidly than if he ate no food at all. This conclusively proves that emaciation is due to the lack of ability on the part of the organism to assimilate the food eaten, rather than to a lack of actual food supplied.*

   —*Hereward Carrington,* Fasting for Health and Long Life

"Food is the greatest producer of disease, and that its proper regulation, as to quality and quantity, is the greatest preventative measure, as well as curative measure, which we know. Why does the athlete always have to go into training for so long a period of time, and take so much exercise in his preparation of any contest requiring endurance? It is simply because his body is in such a condition that this is required, in order to get rid of a lot of useless material which should never have been introduced in the first place. We constantly overeat, and then have to take enforced exercise in order to burn up, and get rid of, this excess of food material! If we did not eat so much in the first place, all this would not be necessary. We should prevent the accumulation of this excess of mal-assimilated food material, and then the toxic or poisonous products which result because of its presence would be avoided." —Hereward Carrington, *Death Deferred*

People overeat for a lot of reasons: boredom, conditioning, habit, false hunger, taste, emotional emptiness. But I think the most common reason, as I've mentioned before, is that the body is not getting the nutrients it needs to feel satiated.

Much of the food available today has too few nutrients, and no matter how much people stuff themselves, they will always desire more because they're not meeting their body's nutritional needs. Think about fast food: A hamburger and fries from the drive-through will certainly fill us up, and because it is so high in calories, it should probably fill us up for an entire day. But it leaves us dissatisfied, and, an hour or so later, we're eating again, just to attain a feeling of satisfaction. Just as someone can starve by not eating enough, people who overeat may be starving for nutrients. And if you're eating low-quality food, you're not only not meeting your body's nutritional needs, you're also creating waste and wasting energy.

If the food you're eating is high in quality, you probably need much less of it than you think you do. High-quality food ensures high-quality health, because it provides the most nutrients with the least amount of waste for the body to process, thus helping the body achieve the formula for health. Raw, ripe, whole, fresh, organic plant foods are the best foods we can possibly eat, because they do exactly that. The best step you can take to attain good health is to reduce the amount of food you consume while eating better-quality foods.

Overeating not only causes a loss of energy and power, it also creates a toxic environment, because excess waste in the digestive tract creates gases that are absorbed into the blood. This toxic load on the bloodstream and our cells will create a lack of oxygen in the blood and a harmful amount of pressure within our cells, which also reduces the oxygen. Otto Warburg, a German biochemist and winner of the 1931 Nobel Prize in Physiology or Medicine, discovered that cancer can live and develop even in the absence of oxygen. Many health writers of the past, such as Arnold Ehret, Hereward Carrington, and St. Louis Estes, have even linked heart disease to excess intestinal gases. In other words, disease can only thrive in a body loaded with a buildup of waste gases from excess amounts of food. We simply pass this off as a harmless burp or fart, but it is the result of the waste in our body trying to get out.

Many other common health problems that result from too much gas in our system include loss of memory, vertigo, eye troubles, depression, hysteria, and even paralysis, where the pressure of the gas building up in our cells is so intense that a large blood vessel gives way. These gases are part of the obstruction we need to avoid to be healthy. Otherwise, they will deplete our system to such an extent that weakness and energy loss will accrue.

> "Most so-called common problems today from nervousness, headaches, poor circulation, cramps, sluggish mentality, acute indigestion, and numerous aches and pains are due to an overload of food in the body which become waste and create gaseous formations in the bowels and stomach."
> —Dr. St. Louis Estes, *Intestinal Flatus or Gas*

When the body doesn't waste energy by trying to metabolize the wrong foods or by having to digest too much food, there will be enough energy left to maintain and build health. It's important to understand the essential factors related to the quality of food and the amount of energy used for digestion. The best foods we can eat are the foods that supply the most nutrition but require the least amount of work for our bodies to digest and assimilate.

## Chew On This

If we overeat any food when our body is already weak, it may be possible that every morsel of food or drink we take in ends up as toxic waste, particularly if we don't chew our food well enough. Chewing is the first stage in digestion, and it is among the most important. The longer and more thoroughly we chew, the easier it will be for our bodies to metabolize our food, and the cleaner we will be internally. Dr. St. Louis Estes states in his book *Raw Food and Health*, "Any kind of food will produce gas in the stomach and bowels if it is not properly masticated." This is why juicing and blending are so helpful.

"Every muscular effort we make, every thought we think, wastes the bodily tissues; they are broken down or destroyed by the effort. This loss is made good by the food we eat, so that to maintain the best possible heath, the equivalence between the 'income' and the 'outgo' should be maintained.

We should eat just enough, not more and not less than is required, to keep the body in this state of physiological equilibrium, 'that just balance we call health.' Less than this amount causes weakness, depletion, exhaustion, loss of weight, and all the symptoms of starvation. More than the required amount has the effect of clogging the body with an excess of effete material and choking and blocking it, and ultimately causing no end of mischief."

—Hereward Carrington

People simply don't chew their food well enough.

# Give It A Rest

We could all be a lot healthier if we would eat when we feel we need food for its value to our well-being and not for emotional reasons. Even then, we should limit our intake to what meets our needs, not what our appetite is clamoring for.

The best way we can stop or prevent overeating is to give our digestive systems a rest. Yes, stop eating for a day or two. This is also known as a fast, or fasting. All the long-time health enthusiasts I have interviewed and whose writings I've studied believe that the secret to health is moderate eating habits and occasional abstinence. I suggest fasting one day a week by consuming only water or green vegetable juices. Almost everyone I know who has tried this has benefited from it, because fasting reduces obstruction and restores energy.

# What Should We Eat?

*The average person has as much as ten pounds of uneliminated feces in the bowels, continually poisoning the bloodstream and the entire system. Every sick person has a more or less mucus-clogged system, such mucus being derived from undigested and uneliminated unnatural food substances, accumulated from childhood on.*
—Arnold Ehret, The Mucusless Diet Healing System

Why don't I advise eating cooked food? Because I believe when food is heated to a temperature above 105 degrees F, many important nutrients, including enzymes, proteins, and vitamins are destroyed. Although it is ideal to eat only raw food, you can begin to reap the benefits of a raw food diet if at least 75 percent of your diet consists of raw food.

When we eat food lacking in enzymes, the body has to expend a tremendous amount of energy digesting the food and then cleansing the body of the accumulated waste. So, when we cook our food, we're actually taking a high-quality food and making it a lower-quality one. Cooking also dries out the food, removing important water and nutritious liquids.

Eating food that is as fresh as possible is also an important part of quality. Once picked, all foods start to lose their nutrients. The longer food sits after being picked, the fewer nutrients it will contain. Chances are the food will be fresher if locally grown, but that's not always the case. Find out when your food was picked, and do your best to eat foods that are as fresh as possible.

Nonorganic, or conventionally grown, food comes from toxic soil, which in turn yields toxic produce. People worry about the quality of water from their tap, but by far the dirtiest water you can ingest, in my opinion, is the water contained in nonorganic fruits and vegetables.

Another reason to eat organic food is because conventional soil is poor in mineral content. Vitamins mostly originate from the sun and elements above the ground, whereas minerals in plants are usually derived from the soil and elements beneath the ground. The quality of food, including its taste, depends largely upon the quality of the soil. This is a reason that simply following a vegetarian or raw food diet doesn't necessarily guarantee high-quality nutrition; the organic factor is an important consideration in what makes a food high quality.

Organic food standards have been under attack for decades by large corporations that want to lower them. So not only is it important to eat organic food for your health, it also is important because every dollar you spend on organic food counts as a vote in its favor. Although organic food sales have grown ten times since 1990, they still don't approach the amount of conventional food sales. Because of the increasing popularity of organic food, even Wal-Mart, the most popular supermarket in the United States, now sells organic products. Consumers of organic food are elated about this, but they are also concerned that big corporations may succeed in lowering organic standards. Whatever happens, buying organic is always preferable to nonorganic, for the health of the consumer and also for the health of the environment.

## Completing the Formula

Until now, I've spoken about the Formula for Health from a nutritional standpoint. However, if you eat the best food in the best way and in the best form but don't take care of your emotional health and wellness, you will still suffer from disease.

Essentially, emotional illness develops when we have more fear than knowledge. This can affect us in minor ways, in the form of just a headache, for example, or we could develop worse conditions, such as anxiety, depression, or even mental illness. All this mental stress is caused by emotional drain. What can we do to keep our emotional state healthy? We can follow the formula for emotional health:

### Knowledge - Fear = Freedom

The more knowledge we have about the causes and cures for disease, the more stable our emotional health will be. When there is a lack of knowledge, doubt sets in. Any combination of confusion or doubt in any area of life will stress the body and can affect us on a physical level.

The paradox of choice is that, when we have too many options, we often choose one that is wrong for us. Many people are tired or exhausted due to poor dietary habits, and when they have too many choices, instead of making a wise choice, they make an easier choice—choosing what's popular. But what's popular is not always what is best for us, and what is best for us is not always popular. Why do we have such an abundance of choices? There are many reasons, but I think the more media we let into our lives, the more information and the more choices we are exposed to.

From my research, I can see there is a single common cause of most of the emotional illnesses afflicting many people today, and it's frightening how many people are addicted to it. I am, of course, referring to television programming and the advertisements we view on TV.

There is a reason why it's called television "programming." Most of the shows on TV overload us with information. When the same information is seen and heard a few times, even if it's not true, people begin to accept it as truth. Many television shows are misleading, presenting a grim, slanted view of reality; the commercials trick us, and the news makes us live in fear. Watching television has many confirmed ill effects. As a result, I think the best way one can achieve the formula for *emotional* health is to

- stop watching television programs, and
- avoid the news.

But, wait a minute—don't we need to know the news to be well-informed citizens? It is my opinion that if something happens that you need to know about, someone will tell you soon enough. Many people watch the news every day and night, filling their minds with fear. In turn, they worry, often without any basis in reality.

My recommendations might seem extreme, but after a short break from television and the news, see how much better you feel. If, for some reason, you don't want to stop watching TV programs or the news, I suggest watching only DVDs for entertainment, and for news, perhaps listen to National Public Radio (NPR), which presents information without that negative twist that can rack us emotionally. Plus, there are many positive news stories on NPR, something you don't often see on television news. Try to take a media or TV fast a few days per week. If you feel you can't get rid of them entirely, or choose not to, at least cut down.

In addition to TV programming and news, another common way we toy with our emotional health is by surrounding ourselves with negative people. The saying goes, "The people you spend most of your time with either become like you, or you become like them." So, chances are, if you're hanging out with negative people, their negative attitude will rub off on you. Try to spend time with people who are positive, upbeat, and optimistic.

These are just the beginning aspects of gaining emotional control. You either control your emotions, or your emotions control you. From an emotional standpoint, people often overeat low-quality foods because they're used to so-called comfort foods. These are the foods people run to when their emotions are out of control. "Emotional eating" often leads to binges of overeating that can become a serious health issue. Foods consumed when emotions are running high are usually of poor quality, and that adds to the problem.

There are many food disorders that may seem, on the surface, to be caused by diet, but the root cause may be emotional. In any stage of disease, it is essential to explore both the emotional and spiritual components. They are as integral to health as the food you eat.

## Formula for Spiritual Heath

The cause of the illness will help us determine the approach for the cure. If we do everything we can physically and emotionally and the problem persists, the trouble might stem from a spiritual issue. There are many words for being spiritual today, and although some people might think all spirituality is the same, there are crucial differences.

It's of utmost importance to thoroughly understand the type of spirituality you are engaged in, because some spiritual beliefs and practices are beneficial and health supporting, while others may be harmful and cause sickness. Let me clarify that being spiritual is not necessarily the same as being religious. I believe being spiritual is having a personal relationship with our Creator. Numerous studies have shown that those who have a strong, supportive, positive spiritual practice tend to be healthier, happier people. The spiritual formula for health is:

## Faith - Doubt = Joy

---

# How to Live to One Hundred and Beyond

One of my greatest inspirations is Luigi Cornaro, an Italian nobleman and playwright who lived between 1464 and 1566. Cornaro lived the charmed life of his class and got away with eating rich food until age thirty-five, when he grew ill. His physician advised him to modify his diet, to eat and drink minimal amounts of food and wine, and to concentrate on those foods that were easiest to digest. He came to realize that no one could know his body better than he could, and eventually he decided to take responsibility for his own health. He observed that overeating clearly was the cause of the long-term health problems of the people around him. He decided to cut back on his food intake.

Cornaro had begun to live what he called the "temperate, moderate, or simple life," which he wrote about in his 1558 book, Trattato de la Vita Sobria, or Treatise on the Simple Life. He ate only twelve ounces a day of solid food, divided into two meals, with fourteen ounces of light wine, also divided into two servings. Within a few months on his new diet, Cornaro's health improved remarkably. Shortly after his new life of wisdom, clarity, and health, he married, had a daughter, and eventually welcomed eleven healthy grandchildren, the joy of his advanced years.

Cornaro believed in consuming the best-quality and most easily digestible foods in small amounts, which is exactly what The Formula for Health prescribes. He enjoyed excellent health on this minimal regimen for forty-five years. He ate a little meat (all cattle were free-range and grass-fed back then), but only in very small portions on special occasions; he would eat one egg yolk, vegetable soup, coarse, unrefined bread, salads, small quantities of locally grown, fresh, seasonal fruits and vegetables, and slightly fermented wine. (It's important to understand that, in those days, wine was not bottled as it is today but was kept in barrels. Since it was consumed the

---

No matter how long it takes and no matter how many times you stumble, stay focused and faithful to a divine plan and your Creator will keep you on the path of health and healing. An obedient heart is the path to health.

---

same year the grapes were harvested, it contained only a fraction of the alcohol found in today's wines.) Neither fish nor chicken agreed with Cornaro, so he avoided them.

At age eighty-five, even though he was happy and satisfied with his diet, his well-meaning relatives were not; they implored him to eat more. Finally, to stop their incessant badgering and to appease them, he increased the amount of his food from twelve to fourteen ounces and his wine from fourteen to sixteen ounces. There were dire consequences; within twelve days, he developed a high fever.

He knew exactly what had caused him to become ill—too much food; so he once again restricted his calorie intake. After three days of smaller meals, his health returned.

At age ninety-five, Luigi Cornaro had all his faculties intact. His judgment, memory, and joyful spirit were undiminished, and he continued a healthy life on small quantities of food and drink. He retained all his senses and had no memory loss—even his eyesight and hearing had grown keener with the years. In his nineties, he studied singing and horseback riding, and, to the end of his days, he led an active life. Until his death, he continued to try to persuade his friends and family of the healthfulness of small meals, and as a perfect guarantee of physical, mental, and emotional happiness.

It's important to note that all food in mid-sixteenth century Europe was of much higher quality than today's commercial fare. It was entirely organic, and there were no packaged foods, no processed foods, and no supplements. None of the plants native to the Americas—coffee, cocoa, tobacco, cane sugar, corn, peanuts, potatoes, tomatoes—had yet been imported. In fact, it wasn't until the nineteenth century that many wealthy Europeans had become addicted to coffee, chocolate, tobacco, and sugar. There were no distilled beverages, no sodas, no processed candies, no white flour and white rice. Natural herbal remedies were the medications most people relied on; there were no petroleum products, no plastics, no factory farming. The world was still truly green, not commercially and environmentally challenged.

# Chapter 4

# Getting the Most from Your Food

So far, we've discussed why we get sick and how food and rest contribute to the vital energy we need for complete wellness. We've learned why we should consume only plant food that is high quality—raw, ripe, fresh, and organic—so that toxins and digestion don't drain our energy. Now let's talk about the important details of a high-quality, raw food diet.

Remember that I said the three main reasons people become interested in health are:

1. To cure disease
2. To prevent disease
3. To stay young looking

A high-quality diet can accomplish all three of these. Having cured myself from a so-called incurable disease and helping others heal as well has changed many of my former beliefs about the important role of nutrition. When I was younger, I foolishly based my beliefs about diet on what was in vogue at time, rather than on the wisdom born of my own experience. Now I know better, and the proof is in the results. Although I am very disciplined and serious about this subject, I've remained open-minded, as I am continually learning more about the relationship between diet and health.

## Habits and Addictions

If you've picked up this book, you most likely know how important diet is to your health. But there are many people who remain in the dark when

it comes to that connection. And there are many people who are aware of the relationship between diet and health yet still have a hard time making the switch to raw, ripe, fresh, organic food, because their lives are often filled with bad habits and addictions.

Let's talk about this for a minute. A habit and an addiction are not the same thing. A habit is something we do on a regular basis, but it is also something we could stop doing if, for example, we found out it's not good for us and we were highly motivated to quit—in other words, we can "break" a habit. But an addiction is something we are compelled to do on a regular basis, something we must do, even when we know it is harmful.

When it comes to eating poor-quality food, we need to change those addictions to habits, and then break them. You *can* do this—with knowledge and discipline. People overcome addictions every day, and go on to create a healthier and more satisfying lifestyle for themselves.

Of all the addictions we hear about today, unhealthful dietary habits top the list as the most common. I should know; I was very addicted to unhealthful food, and I suffered as a result. I am happy to report that I overcame those addictions a long time ago, and I am never tempted to revisit my unwise choices. I am confident that, with a wise plan and discipline, anyone can have victory over their struggles with food addictions, just as I have.

To overcome addictions, we need to understand and have faith in the great healing powers of the human body, seek our Creator for wisdom, and find support from friends and family. Physical healing from any health challenge needs to be accompanied by natural methods, such as herbs, food, rest, sunlight, exercise, and fresh air. Then, just let the body do the job it was designed to do.

# Understanding Your Food

All food is made up of three macronutrients: protein, carbohydrates, and fat. There are healthful choices in all of these categories, but eating one to the exclusion of all others can be harmful. Fortunately, most foods contain all three in varying amounts.

## Proteins

Proteins are an important part of every living cell. They are necessary for growth, development, and cellular repair. A source of heat and energy, proteins also aid in the formation of hormones, enzymes, and antibodies, while maintaining the body's acid-alkaline balance.

To make proteins available, the body breaks down large protein molecules into simpler units called amino acids. There are two types of amino acids: essential and nonessential. The body produces nonessential amino acids, but essential amino acids must be obtained through food because the body cannot create them. There are eight essential amino acids, all of which can be found in a vegetarian diet. Bee pollen, soybeans, hempseeds, and some berries are a few of the vegetarian sources that contain all eight amino acids and are therefore called "complete" proteins.

Most people in the Western world eat far too much protein, largely due to a diet high in meat and dairy products. Eating too much protein results in physical imbalances that may present, for example, as kidney problems or colon cancer. These ailments lead people to their doctors, who typically prescribe drugs to deal with the harmful effects of the problem. Taking drugs is not the cure; the cure is to stop overeating animal products and other high-protein foods, such as nuts, fortified protein drinks, protein powders, and "energy" bars. Eat a raw, ripe, fresh, organic diet and your health will improve.

# Fats

The body does need certain fats to thrive, especially during infancy and childhood. They are important for brain development, and they provide energy and support growth. After the first two years of life, an infant's fat requirements drop to only small amounts. But today, people continue to consume fat throughout their lives, and they consume way too much. Excessive fat intake is a major contributor to obesity, high blood pressure, heart disease, and colon cancer, just to name a few of the illnesses it is responsible for.

Nature gives us healthful fats contained in raw plant foods, such as nuts, seeds, avocados, coconuts, olives, akees (a tropical fruit native to West Africa), and durians (a tropical fruit native to Southeast Asia). There are also many other plant foods that are lesser-known but excellent sources of fat. In fact, raw purslane, a wild, edible weed commonly grown on most lawns, has more omega-3 fatty acids than fish oil. Such natural fats are healthful and the body needs them to thrive. Be sure to eat a good variety to ensure that you don't miss out on the different types.

On the downside, there are fats that come from natural sources that are transformed into deadly substances through commercial processing, including animal and plant fats, such as cooking oils. These processed fats and the foods that contain them or are cooked in them will eventually cause disease, slowing you down by clogging the blood vessels. If you abuse your body with an addiction to harmful fatty foods, you are certain to face illness sooner or later. Food that is altered from its natural state is dangerous to our health. If we accept the foods given by nature, in the form they are naturally provided, we will enjoy far superior health.

## Carbohydrates

Today, everyone is concerned about carbohydrates. Many people don't realize that there are different types of carbohydrates, and some, such as low-sugar fruits, are perfectly all right, while others, such as refined white flour, can be as bad for us as everybody says they are.

Simple carbohydrates are sugars, both artificial and naturally occurring. They are found in various syrups, sweeteners, processed foods, and dairy products, as well as in fruits and nonstarchy vegetables.

Foods such as bread, legumes, rice, pasta, and starchy vegetables contain complex carbohydrates. In my opinion, complex carbohydrates are the foods we'd do best to avoid. They are very challenging for the body to process and therefore are not healthful. Eating too many complex carbohydrates can cause discomfort and disease. They make the body work very hard to digest them, and during that process they are converted to sugar, or glucose, in the body, leading to blood sugar problems. It's a smart idea to avoid or at least cut down on the amount of complex carbohydrates in your diet.

## Sugars

Sugars are tricky. We know that processed sugar is not good for us, but because of our addictions, we continue to consume foods that contain it. This is an emotional issue and is not due to a lack of knowledge. What many people do not realize is that natural sugars can be just as harmful as white sugar. Natural sugars are in many foods, particularly fruits. Fruit is a completely healthful and nutritious food in its ripe, raw, organic, natural state, but when it is hybridized and/or processed, it is no longer a good choice for us.

Today, we have seedless fruits that contain more sugar and fewer nutrients than ever before. Manufacturers also take delicious whole fruit, juice it, pasteurize it, add tons of sugar to it, and call it "fruit juice," when in reality it is a cheap, low-quality form of a high-quality food. It is important to get nutrients straight from their whole, natural source, because, the more they are processed or tampered with, the more harmful they become to our body.

Regardless of the type of sugar you consume, too much of it can cause problems. Excess sugar causes fermentation that feeds and promotes yeast growth and feeds harmful bacteria in the body. This fermentation also creates gas and forms the basis for many diseases—from candida to cancer and everything in between. If you want to be healthy, you must cut back on sugary and starchy foods. And, without question, you must cut out all processed sugars.

## The Chew-Chew Train

One of the key elements of the Formula for Health that I talked about in chapter 3 is to use as little energy as possible for digestion. When you're eating only healthful foods, that's doable. Another way to conserve energy that would otherwise be used for digestion is to chew your food well. Digestion begins in the mouth, and if we grind our food into a liquid before we swallow it, we create even less work for our digestive system and make it easier for the body to extract the nutrients from our food. Chewing, or mastication, stimulates the salivary glands to release saliva, which begins to act on the food immediately, breaking it down before it even makes its way to the stomach.

I've already discussed how overeating drains our energy. There is yet another reason why overeating is harmful. Consuming a large amount of food without chewing it sufficiently spells trouble for the intestines, as it is very difficult to digest and assimilate the nutrients from large chunks of food.

There is no guideline indicating how long you should chew your food, although, in the 1800s, natural health advocates had many discussions and requirements about this in their writings and lectures. To be on the safe side, the simplest rule to follow is to always chew your food thoroughly, until it is as smooth, creamy, and liquid as possible.

If the thought of all that chewing wears you out, or if you just need an occasional break from it, there are other ways to enjoy a healthful diet that don't require so much "work"—juicing and blending. Both of these preparation methods can save your body some energy with both chewing and digesting. There is a saying I like to use that explains it well: chew your drinks, and drink your food.

Juicing is extracting the juices from fruits, vegetables, grasses, and sprouts in a juicer, which is a machine that separates the food's juice, or liquid, from the fiber, or pulp. While there is absolutely nothing wrong with the pulp—it contains many important phytonutrients in addition to fiber—the point of juicing is to give your body a rest from the chewing and digestive activity while still getting most of the nutrients from the food.

The juice of fresh, organic produce is packed with vitamins, minerals, enzymes, amino acids, and natural sugars. It also supplies valuable electrolytes and oxygen to the cells for use in cleansing and rebuilding.

Please don't mistake coffee, tea, cow's milk, and carbonated and artificially sweetened soda as healthful beverages. They are devoid of all nutrients, are acid forming, and will create a tremendous obstruction, or energy loss, in your body. Beverages from natural sources, such as fresh fruit and vegetable juices and nut and seed milks, prepared at home, not prepackaged, are far more healthful choices.

Another way to get complete nutrition while using as little energy as possible is to consume blended foods. An example of a blended food is raw soup made by processing lettuce and/or several vegetables together in a blender.

The major difference between juicing and blending is that blending retains the fiber. The digestive system will have far less work to do to digest and assimilate blended food than if you chewed the food. By blending your food, you can offset insufficient chewing. You will receive all the nutritional benefits, and the food is already prepared for absorption and assimilation.

Another caveat: don't consider commercially prepared puddings or gelatins as healthful. Your blended diet should consist of only the highest quality foods available: raw, ripe, fresh, and organic fruits, vegetables, nuts, seeds, and live foods, such as sprouts.

Use mostly vegetables in your juices and blended foods. You may mix small amounts of fruit with the vegetables, such as an apple to sweeten a green vegetable juice, but the bulk of the juice should be vegetables, or, at the most, fruits that are low in sugar, such as blueberries, blackberries, green apples, cucumber, and zucchini. Even if you are consuming 100 percent juice from a low-sugar fruit, it is a good idea to add at least 50 to 75 percent water to lessen the rush of sugar into the bloodstream.

Juicing is not necessarily better than blending, or blending better than juicing; it depends on the goal. I think juicing and blending are more healthful than eating foods in their whole state because most people don't chew thoroughly or properly. If people actually chewed their food the way they should, it wouldn't make too much difference whether it was blended, juiced, or consumed whole; in fact, it's likely that eating the whole food would be best. The most important dietary consideration after quality and quantity is variety. Include an assortment of foods, with a balanced combination of juiced, blended, and whole raw vegetables and fruits.

## Food Combining

Another great way to conserve energy is to eat foods in an order and a combination that facilitates digestion. This is known as food combining.

Mixing the wrong foods together or eating them in the wrong order can sap energy and cause systemic fermentation and putrification of the food.

Food combining is a way to eat that allows for easier digestion and minimal digestive conflicts. It works like this: Every food takes a certain amount of time to digest. Eating similar foods with similar digestive times helps the body digest meals more easily; these foods are said to combine well. For example, watermelon takes about one hour to digest; almonds may take up to five hours. In view of this, eating watermelon and almonds at the same meal is not a good idea—it's known as a poor combination. Eating too many meals like this may cause constipation, bloating, and gas, which may lead to more serious issues.

Since there are different types of raw food, each with its unique digestive time, your body will have to work harder to digest foods eaten in poor combinations. Ideally, your body will use as little power as possible for digestion—the very reason it's important to combine your foods properly. In general, it helps to eat liquid foods with other liquid foods, and dense foods with other dense foods. I suggest reading some of the books written on food combining to learn as much as you can.

## How food combining works

Fred Bisci, a long-time raw foodist, has been studying diet and nutrition for more than fifty years. I have followed his recommendations for food combining for years. Here is his explanation of food combining:

- There are three basic types of food: concentrated food (proteins and carbohydrates), food with a high water content (fruits and vegetables), and fats.
- Proteins are the most complex (concentrated) food and require the most time and energy to digest and assimilate.
- Fruit is the least complex food (with the highest water content) and takes the least amount of time and energy to digest and assimilate. It

can be eaten right before, but not after, any other food. After a meal, wait at least three hours before eating more fruit.

- Glucose (sugar) is the brain's primary food, so the brain needs mostly carbohydrates.
- Most fruit passes through the stomach and into the intestines in about forty-five minutes; dried fruit, bananas, and avocados take longer.

I think medical science and nutritionists have erroneously classified all sugars, including fruit, as carbohydrates. Fruit may be technically classified as a carbohydrate, but its makeup is so entirely different that it should be thought of as a separate group. In my opinion, it is best to classify fruit as a sugar. Because most people wrongly think of fruit as a carbohydrate, they subsequently consume it along with proteins, and this has probably led to more digestive difficulties than any other dietary habit.

In the digestive system, the processes that break down proteins, carbohydrates, and fruit are entirely different, requiring different secretions. Therefore, to ensure the most efficient digestion possible, don't eat these three types of foods in the same meal.

Avoid eating proteins with carbohydrates (such as cooked beans and potatoes), proteins with high-sugar carbohydrates (such as nuts and raisins), or complex carbohydrates with high-sugar carbohydrates (such as cooked grain cereal with apple or banana). The different digestive juices coming in contact will nullify each other's effectiveness, causing the protein to putrefy and the carbohydrate to ferment. The result is gas and flatulence.

- Proteins (concentrated foods) should be eaten with steamed vegetables and/or salads (foods with a high water content) for optimum digestion.
- Carbohydrates (concentrated foods) should be eaten with steamed vegetables and/or salads (foods with a high water content) for optimum digestion.

- If fruit is eaten alone on an empty stomach, it will have the effect of washing and cleaning the digestive tract, leaving it more capable of absorbing nutrients.

- Always eat spinach raw. Spinach contains oxalic acid, which assists in the peristaltic action of the digestive system, the constant "waving" motion that keeps food moving through it. When cooked, oxalic acid is transformed into acid crystals in the kidneys and its beneficial properties are lost.

- To get the most out of tomatoes, always eat them raw. Tomatoes are an acid fruit, but in the digestive tract, raw tomatoes are extremely alkaline, helping neutralize acid buildup in the body.

  When tomatoes are cooked, they become highly acid-forming and damaging to the internal organs. They are a prime factor in the high incidence of ulcers in the United States and will severely aggravate an existing ulcer. If you must have cooked tomatoes (as in spaghetti sauce), eat a large green salad at the same time to offset the damaging effects.

- Do not drink water or any beverages during or immediately after a meal. Fluids wash away and dilute many of the digestive juices. This forces the body to immediately secrete more digestive juices, usurping your vital energy.

- Avoid dairy products. They are highly mucus-forming and difficult to digest. They do not combine well with anything.

By adhering to the rules of proper food combining, the digestive system is given less work, thereby conserving energy that can then be utilized elsewhere in the body or for clearing out accumulated waste and toxins.

Improper food combining is one of the main reasons so many people are overweight. The energy required to break down and eliminate excess food is constantly being used by the digestive system. There is simply not enough energy at the body's disposal to carry out the digestive processes.

Ignore fad weight-loss schemes and standardized height/weight charts based on averages from an unhealthy population. The critical point to remember is when you are on a nutritious, vital diet, your body will automatically return to your optimum weight and will remain there.

## Sequential Eating

Stanley Bass, a natural hygiene doctor in New York, taught me another wise way to consume food called *sequential eating*. Sequential eating is similar to food combining, but instead of combinations, sequential eating focuses on consuming one food at a time, It advocates eating the most easily digested foods first and denser foods last. This is also referred to as *layered eating*—a simple and wise way to eat.

Consuming one food at a time ensures the greatest possible ease of digestion. A group of research scientists at Columbia University has found evidence that a meal is digested in the exact order it is eaten—one food group at a time, regardless of its complexity or quantity. According to the practice of sequential eating, if you start with a relatively concentrated food that takes a long time to break down, followed by a food that takes only half that time, digestion of the second food will be delayed, and it will start to ferment and decompose before it can be digested, losing much of its nutritional value.

Both proper food combining and sequential eating are excellent ways to eat and offer a tremendous advantage over the standard way most people consume their meals. Of course, there will always be some people who can mix their foods and not have problems. But many can't, so I recommend heeding correct food-combining rules, and, if possible, sequential eating. I suggest printing and placing the following food-combining chart on your refrigerator door.

# Food Combining Chart

ACID FRUITS: Eat with green, nonstarchy vegetables and before other fruits.

Blackberries
Grapefruit
Lemon
Lime
Orange
Pineapple
Raspberries
Strawberries
Tangerines
Tomatoes

LOWER-ACID FRUITS: Eat with green, nonstarchy vegetables.

Apple
Apricot
Blueberries
Cherimoya
Cherries
Fresh figs
Grapes
Kiwifruit
Mango
Nectarine
Papaya
Peach
Pear
Plums

SWEET FRUIT: Eat with green, nonstarchy vegetables.

Bananas
Dates
Dried fruit/raisins

Persimmon
Thompson and Muscat grapes

MELON: Do not eat with other fruit. Eat with green, nonstarchy vegetables.

Canataloupe
Casaba
Crane
Crenshaw
Honeydew
Persian
Sharlyn
Watermelon

PROTEIN: Eat with nonstarchy vegetables.

Coconut
Nuts
Olives
Seeds

OILY FRUIT: Do not eat with Protein or any Fruit.

Avocado

CARBOHYDRATES: Eat with Oily Fruit, Nonstarchy or Mildly Starchy Vegetables. Do not eat with Fruit.

Potatoes
Squash

NONSTARCHY VEGETABLES: Eat with any food.

Asparagus

Bell peppers
Broccoli
Brussels sprouts
Cabbage
Celery
Chard
Collard
Cucumber
Eggplant
Endive
Green beans
Kale
Kohlrabi
Lettuce
Parsley
Spinach
Turnips
Zucchini

MILDLY STARCHY VEGETABLES: Do not eat with Protein.

Artichokes
Beets
Carrots
Cauliflower
Corn
Peas

Do not eat:

Animal products, soybeans

Not recommended:

Beans, grains, grain products, bread, cereals, pasta, garlic, leeks, onions, radishes, scallions, shallots

# Getting the Worst from Your Food

*Every microwave oven leaks electromagnetic radiation, harms food, and converts substances cooked in it to dangerous organ-toxic and carcinogenic products.*
—Lita Lee, *Health Effects of Microwave Radiation*

One of the saddest things I see when traveling is widespread addiction to low-quality food. People are choosing more and more to prepare their food in microwave ovens, forgoing high quality for convenience. This is one of the most harmful things you can do, yet people do it every day. I shudder to think that just about every North American home today has a microwave oven.

It's bad enough that people who are not interested in health use microwave ovens, but it's even sadder when people who profess to be concerned about health use them, unaware of the harm they cause. Recently, I was reading a popular health magazine that featured an article that encouraged microwaving to save time. It spoke of all the delicious recipes that can be prepared quickly and easily in a microwave oven.

I think that it's not just the preparation of food in a microwave oven that is harmful, but the radiation the food is exposed to. In my opinion, merely heating water in the microwave, instead of boiling it on the stove, makes the water toxic.

Did you know that in 1976 the Soviet Union banned the use of microwave ovens because they understood the harm that might be caused from eating food cooked in them? Scientific evidence now confirms that microwave ovens produce cancer-causing effects in food, in addition to the destruction of nutrients. There are so many harmful issues with microwave ovens that I could write a book on that subject alone. Many concerned writers already have, and the information is gradually becoming more available to the public through books, articles, and the

Internet. Microwaved food robs more energy from the body than any other method of food preparation because microwaving changes the food's molecules into unnatural forms. Microwaving also robs food of minerals, vitamins, and other nutrients so that the body gets little or no benefit from the food, or the body absorbs these altered compounds, which cannot be broken down.

## Those Killer Fried Foods

Another harmful way to prepare food that so many people today chose is frying. When I was a teenager, I'd get a stomachache and pimples on my face every time I ate fried food. Before I'd eat a slice of my then-beloved pizza, I would sop up the floating grease on top of each slice with a napkin. Years later, I learned how horrific fried foods are to our health. The scary thing is that most people know this but still continue to consume fried foods. Unlike microwave ovens, for which the case reports and studies are not common knowledge, the news regarding fried foods has been public information for many years. How frightening it is that just about everybody knows how dangerous it is to eat fried foods, yet people still won't stop eating them or even cut down on them. Are fleeting taste sensations more important than long-term health?

Do your best to avoid all harmful foods, but make sure to give special attention to avoiding the worst foods—those that are microwaved and fried.

## Other Health Destroyers

It's important to note that in addition to overindulging, eating unhealthful foods, and using harmful food preparation methods, there are other habits you may have that are equally as harmful to your health and will waste your energy. Although these are not the main focus of this book, they are just as important to avoid if you desire good health:

- Negative thoughts and emotions (such as stress, worry, fear, anger, and anxiety)
- Alcohol and drugs
- Misuse of sexual energy

Any of these have the potential to create disease, and, as with overeating, they are pervasive in today's diseased world. Remember, we are whole human beings. We can't expect to be healthy simply by changing our diet; we have to consider these other lifestyle factors and habits as well.

## To Supplement or Not

It's important to try to get all our nutrients from food. Every known nutrient the body needs to thrive can be found in fruits and vegetables, and that is the first place we should try to get them. If, for some reason, we are not able to get all the needed nutrients that way, supplements can help us stay healthy.

There are several reasons that we might not be able to obtain all our nutrients from food:
- Our food may be low quality.
- We may not be eating a sufficient variety of foods.
- We may have absorption or assimilation problems.

For any of these cases, supplementation can be the solution. I only suggest a few supplements that I'm confident will help most people either improve or maintain their health: digestive enzymes, probiotics, green superfood powders (I like the Synergy brand), and liquid algae (E-3 Live). Other than these supplements, I suggest finding out what might be best for you. (I will discuss this more in chapter 5.)

## Nutrition Wrap-Up

There is no "right" way to health for everyone, because we are all starting out from different points. We learn about healthful eating at different times in our lives, and we've all created different levels of illness that we must overcome. There are many variables to determine what will work best for our own individual chemistry and lifestyle, so the exact treatment will be unique for each person. Having said that, though, I do believe there are some standard guidelines that will benefit everyone.

The human body is designed to eat, digest, and assimilate certain foods more easily than others. However, it can adapt to accept all foods and appear to be just fine, at least for a certain amount of time. Just because we are unaware of the pain our diet and lifestyle are causing doesn't mean disease is not taking place.

The highest-quality foods for our health and healing are raw, fresh, and organic ripe fruits, vegetables, nuts, seeds, and live foods. They are the most easily digested and nutrient-dense foods, and they keep our bodies clean. Overly processed, nonorganic food will cause problems in the long run.

From a health and nutrition standpoint, there is absolutely no need or reason to consume animal products. Every known nutrient can be found in plant foods, without the toxic load that animal flesh leaves in the body. A vegetarian diet also favors the environment, because less land is needed to produce the food.

Remember that the most common causes of disease are overeating and insufficient sleep. To maintain our health, all food should be limited to our nutritional needs. More energy is used by digestion than any other activity, so the more we eat, the more energy we need, and the more sleep we require.

Whatever your experiences with diet and health have been in the past, I want you to know that you can start over with a fresh way of thinking. You will see results. You can be successful on this plan. Let's get started.

# Chapter 5

# Four Steps to Better Health

At my lectures, I meet many people who have chosen my formula for health but who still can't seem to achieve the level of wellness they're after. One thing or another seems to stymie them along the way, and they lose sight of their direction. Because of this, I've devised a simple, four-step process to help people overcome disease:

1. Eliminate the cause of the problem.
2. Cleanse and heal from the damage that was done in the past.
3. Create a diet and lifestyle based on your own personal chemistry.
4. Grow in emotional and spiritual stability.

## Step One: Eliminate the Cause

Many people eat a very poor diet, but because of their lack of understanding about health, they don't even realize it. Or they overeat and continue to get sicker and sicker with every passing day because of their excessive yet insufficient diet. Or they begin cleansing and even may add some healthful foods to their diet, but it's counterproductive to keep eating unhealthful foods while adding good ones. (Remember that health doesn't begin with what you *add* to your diet, but with what you *leave out*, so the first step toward regaining health is to eliminate the unhealthful foods, not just add the good ones.) It's true that eating healthfully is beneficial no matter what, but discontinuing the health-defeating behavior is the first step to becoming well.

In terms of nutrition, the body can't tell the difference between one food and another. All it looks for in food is nutrients: vitamins, minerals,

65

amino acids, enzymes, and so forth. It takes what it needs and then has to get rid of the rest.

Leaving very little waste for our bodies to deal with is the key when it comes to good health. Of course, giving the body the nutrients it needs is important also, but getting those nutrients from sources that won't use massive amounts of our essential power and energy to digest them is the answer. A steak might provide a small amount of nutrients the body can use, but it will also leave a substantial amount of waste for the body to contend with. An apple, though, has many nutrients but little waste. This is why juicing and blending are so important: they enable you to consume foods that are partially "digested." The body easily assimilates all the nutrients and doesn't have to work hard to get rid of the waste.

It's also important to keep in mind that there are factors that can cause nutrient deficiencies, which also can contribute to illness. For instance, nutrients, whether they're amino acids, vitamins, minerals, or enzymes, all work synergistically. If we're missing one, it usually will affect the absorption of another. For example, an insufficient intake of vitamins and minerals, especially vitamin C, can interfere with the absorption of amino acids. And if you've not been eating a healthful diet in the past, you could also have lost some ability to adequately absorb nutrients.

The amount of nutrients each person needs will vary with the individual. Most people overconsume, and more is not necessarily better. What the body can't use, it has to get rid of.

Disease is either a deficiency or detoxification, but most often it is a combination of both of these—getting too few nutrients along with producing and eliminating too much waste. Many people think they're getting too little from their food when in fact they're getting too much.

The more toxic or "unclean" your body is, the more you might feel the continuous need to eat. If you feel sick when you go without food, that's a sign that your body is cleansing itself and an indication that you probably need less food, not more. You may feel better if you eat, but only because you've temporarily stopped the body's natural cleansing process. The cleaner the body is internally, and the higher the quality of your diet, the less food you will need to consume, because your body will be getting so many more nutrients from the food you do eat.

The first habit we should eliminate to gain health, as I discussed previously, is overeating. The next step is to avoid what I call the Top Five Worst Foods.

## Meat

In Western cultures, we are programmed from a very early age to believe that we must eat meat to be healthy. That couldn't be more incorrect.

There are many reasons not to eat meat. As I've mentioned before, meat might provide a small amount of nutrients, but the tremendous amount of waste remaining is very harmful and saps your energy as your body tries to deal with and eliminate it. Meat contains all of the hormones, antibiotics, and other chemicals that the animal was given; these are passed on to you when you eat meat. Eating meat has been linked to many diseases, including cancer. Meat is also extremely acid forming, disrupting the body's delicate acid-alkaline balance.

Today, there is absolutely no reason for people to eat meat and other animal products. A vegan diet is capable of supplying all of our vital nutrients, while leaving the least amount of waste. Please don't be fooled into thinking that fish is a better choice over other types of meats. Fish can be laden with heavy metals and can pass on diseases from polluted water.

## Soda

Probably the most common beverages consumed to excess today are sodas and other soft drinks. These drinks are loaded with sugar, dyes, and chemicals that may lead directly to disease. Did you know that if you put soda in the tailpipe of a car it will destroy the rust? Now think about what it's doing to the inside of your body when you drink it! Diet soda is just as bad, if not worse. There are many studies showing diet soda to be even more acid-forming and more toxic to the body than regular soda.

## Dirty Water

The cleanest water you can find is in organic, living food. The most harmful water is found in nonorganic, or conventionally grown, fruits and vegetables. But the most commonly consumed dirty water comes from the tap. Tap water and water from nonorganic foods can be loaded with many drugs and harmful chemicals. The chlorinated and fluoridated water most people drink today from their municipal water supplies can be, over time, very harmful to the body. To make matters worse, chemical poisons used in farming and those from chemical spills and dumps make our water even deadlier.

A home water filter, preferably an ionized water filter, will help; but even more helpful would be to drink spring water from a source you know is pure and natural. Try them all and use the one you think is best, but avoid tap water.

## Sugar

Sugar is the most widely consumed harmful food. There are many forms of sugar. Refined white sugar and high-fructose corn syrup are highly processed and the most harmful. Overeating any type of sugar is deadly. Sugar ferments faster than any other substance. This fermentation produces gases, and if these gases don't exit the body, they back up into the bloodstream, feeding and promoting yeast growth and harmful bacteria, causing disease over time. All candida, yeast, and harmful molds, collectively known as *microforms*, multiply as we consume more sugar. Gabriel

Cousens, in his book *Rainbow Green Live-Food Cuisine*, said it best: "Sugar feeds negative microforms like gasoline feeds a fire."

Sugar is everywhere today, and not just where you would expect it. Starch in potatoes, pasta, or bread converts to sugar in the body. People are always surprised to learn that eating a baked potato has the same effect on your blood sugar as a soda. The body does need sugar to thrive, of course, but those sugars should come from fresh, organic fruits, only in moderation, and always eaten with the skin or peel, which helps regulate your blood sugar.

Many health enthusiasts believe that all fruits are fine to eat because they have natural sugars in them. Your body does not differentiate between "natural" sugars and any other kind. Sugar is sugar, whether it's from a pear or a Pepsi. Bacteria and yeasts love it and will use it to create a toxic environment in your body.

Unripe fruit also tends to make the body acidic. When the body becomes too acidic, and has the added health pressures resulting from bacteria and yeast, oxygen is prevented from being available to the cells and tissues.

I suggest avoiding all fruits that are high in sugar and limiting the low-sugar fruits. The chart on page 70 is an excellent guide to acceptable foods that contain sugar, based on the glycemic index.

The glycemic index (GI) ranks carbohydrates on a scale of 0 to 100 according to their effect on blood glucose levels after they're consumed. Foods with a high GI number are those that are quickly digested and cause high fluctuations in blood sugar. Those with a low GI number are more slowly digested and produce more gradual rises in blood sugar and insulin levels.

High GI foods—those with a number above 70—should be eaten sparingly because they can elevate blood sugar and lead to minor problems,

# Glycemic Index Ranges

Low: less than 56   Medium: between 56 and 69   High: greater than 69

**BEANS**
baby lima 32
baked 43
black 30
brown 38
butter 31
chickpeas 33
kidney 27
lentil 30
navy 38
pinto  42
red lentils 27
split peas 32
soy 18

**BREADS**
bagel 72
croissant 67
Kaiser roll   73
pita 57
pumpernickel 49
rye  64
rye, dark 76
rye, whole 50
white 72
whole wheat 72
waffles 76

**CEREALS**
All Bran 44
Bran Chex 58
Cheerios 74
Corn Bran 75
Corn Chex 83
Cornflakes 83
Cream of Wheat 66
Crispix 87
Frosted Flakes 55
Grapenuts 67
Grapenuts Flakes 80

Life 66
muesli 60
NutriGrain 66
oatmeal 49
oatmeal, instant 66
puffed wheat 74
puffed rice 90
rice bran 19
Rice Chex 89
Rice Krispies 82
Shredded Wheat 69
Special K 54
Swiss Muesli 60
Team 82
Total 76

**COOKIES**
graham crackers 74
oatmeal 55
shortbread 64
vanilla wafers 77

**CRACKERS**
Kavli Norwegian 71
rice cakes 82
rye 63
saltine 72
stoned wheat thins 67
water crackers 78

**DESSERTS**
angel food cake 67
banana bread 47
blueberry muffin 59
bran muffin 60
Danish 59
fruit bread 47
pound cake  54
sponge cake 46

**FRUIT**
apple 38

apricot, canned 64
apricot, dried 30
apricot jam 55
banana 62
banana, unripe 30
cantaloupe 65
cherries 22
dates, dried 103
fruit cocktail 55
grapefruit 25
grapes 43
kiwi 52
mango 55
orange 43
papaya 58
peach 42
pear 36
pineapple 66
plum 24
raisins 64
strawberries 32
strawberry jam 51
watermelon 72

**GRAINS**
barley 72
brown rice 66
buckwheat 54
bulger 47
chickpeas 36
cornmeal 68
couscous 65
hominy 40
millet 75
rice, instant 91
rice, parboiled 47
rye 34
sweet corn 55
wheat, whole 41
white rice 88

wh. rice, high amylose
   59

**JUICES**
agave nector 11
apple 41
grapefruit 48
orange 55
pineapple 46

**MILK PRODUCTS**
chocolate milk 34
ice cream 50
milk 34
pudding 43
soy milk 31
yogurt 38

**PASTA**
brown rice pasta 92
gnocchi 68
linguine, durum 50
macaroni 46
macaroni & cheese 64
spaghetti 40
spag. prot. enrich. 28
vermicelli 35
vermicelli, rice 58

**SWEETS**
honey 58
jelly beans 80
Life Savers 70
M&M's Choc. Peanut
   33
Skittles 70
Snickers 41

*For a more complete list please search the internet or read the book The New Glucose Revolution: The Authoritative Guide to the Glycemic Index - the Dietary Solution for Lifelong Health (Glucose Revolution) by Dr. Jennie Brand-Miller, Thomas M.S. Wolever, Kaye Foster-Powell, and Stephen Colagiuri (Paperback - Dec 6, 2006) such as drowsiness and fatigue, and to more serious problems, such as hypoglycemia, diabetes, and heart disease. Low GI foods—those below 55—are generally considered more healthful. Those between 55 and 70 are in the intermediate category and should not be eaten often.

Because high GI fruits are so sweet, they can be addictive, and there is a strong tendency to eat too many of them. You should limit all dried fruits—pineapple, bananas, apricots, cantaloupe, dates, kiwifruit, orange juice, grapefruit juice, and mangoes.

On page 72 is an excellent chart by Dr. Cousens, from his book *Rainbow Green Live-Food Cuisine*, which he has permitted me to use to describe the best foods to avoid in three stages for optimal health.

For additional information about the glycemic index, I recommend reading *The New Glucose Revolution: The Authoritative Guide to the Glycemic Index* by Jennie Brand-Miller (Marlowe and Company 2006). For more information about which foods to limit because of their high sugar content, I would suggest reading *The pH Miracle* by Robert O. Young and Shelley Redford Young (Warner Books 2003) and *Rainbow Green Live-Food Cuisine* by Gabriel Cousens (North Atlantic Books 2003). While there are other useful and informative books on the subject, these three cover the subject well.

## Flour

Flours are ground grains. Whole grain flours contain the bran and germ of the grain, but white flour has been stripped of the bran and germ and is then bleached. Although we are led to believe that whole wheat products are good for us, they are still quite processed. Think of processed flour as another form of sugar. Flour products quickly convert to sugar in the bloodstream. This makes starchy food made with flour a poor choice for those in search of health.

# Summary of Food Phases

*From Rainbow Green Live-Food Cuisine by Gabreal Cousins

| Phase 1 | Phase 1.5 | Phase II | Phase II (Minimal Use) | Rainbow Green Live-Food Cuisine Foods to Avoid |
|---|---|---|---|---|
| Nuts & Seeds | Coconut water (diluted with other ingredients) | Yams (raw) | Yams (cooked) | All processed foods |
| Coconut pulp | | Sweet potatoes (raw) | Sweet potatoes (cooked) | |
| All greens | | Pumpkin (raw) | Pumpkin (cooked) | All animal products: |
| All vegetables (except those listed elsewhere) | Carrots (raw) | Parsnips (raw) | Parsnips (cooked) | Flesh |
| | Hard squash (raw) | Beets (raw) | Beets (cooked) | Dairy |
| | Grapefruit | Rutabaga (raw) | Rutabaga (cooked) | Eggs |
| Summer squash (raw) zucchini, patti pan, yellow summer squash | Raspberries | Oranges | Hard squash (cooked) | All grains (except those listed) |
| | Blueberries | Apples | | |
| | Strawberries | Pears | Summer squash (cooked) | Corn |
| | Cherries | Peaches | | |
| Sea vegetables | Cranberries (fresh, unsweetened) | Plums | Straight carrot juice | White potatoes |
| Tomatoes | | Pomegranates | Straight orange juice | White rice |
| Avocados | Goji berries | Blackberries | High-glycemic fruits: | White flour |
| Cucumber | Low-glycemic Tree of Life mesquite meal | Grapefruit juice (diluted with water) | Apricots | Honey |
| Red bell pepper | | | Figs | Sugar |
| Flax oil | | | Grapes | Alcohol |
| Hemp oil | Non-stored grains: | Raw carob | Raisins | Coffee |
| Olive oil | Wild rice | Bee pollen | Melons | Caffeine |
| Sesame oil | Quinoa | | Mangos | Tobacco |
| Almond oil | Buckwheat | Unfermented soy products (as a transition food) | Bananas | Heated oil (except coconut oil) |
| Sunflower oil | Millet | | Papaya | |
| Coconut oil (butter) | Amaranth | | Pineapple | |
| Lemons | Spelt | | Kiwi | Soy sauce & nama Shoyu |
| Limes | Fermented Foods: | | Sapote | |
| Klamath Lake algae (e-3 live) | Apple cider vinegar | | Cherimoya | Yeast |
| | Miso | | Rambutian | Brewer's yeast |
| Super green powders | Sauerkraut | | Durian | Nutritional yease |
| | Kefir | | Dates | Mushrooms |
| Stevia | | | Dried fruits | Peanuts |
| | | | Fresh, raw, fruit juices | Cashews |
| | | | Seed cheese | Cottonseed |
| | | | Cooked, organic, whole foods | Bottled juices |

Most people are under the impression that they're supposed to eat grains and other flour products, but grains today are not the same as they were in the past; the majority have been genetically modified. Most grain products are also highly processed, so what was once passable is no longer safe.

Wheat flour also contains gluten, and several diseases today are associated with gluten in the diet, including inflammatory bowel disease and celiac disease.

## Step Two: Cleanse and Heal

Once you've eliminated all the harmful foods from your diet, you can now begin to clean and rebuild from the damage that was caused before you adopted the Formula for Health. Many people, even those who eat an excellent diet, need to cleanse or they may end up dealing with some sort of health challenge. There are several ways to cleanse and rebuild; although these are two different functions, when the body is cleansing, it is rebuilding at the same time.

Nobel Prize winner Alexis Carrel was able to keep tissue cells alive indefinitely. By supplying needed nutrients and clearing away waste, not only did the cells survive, they also showed no signs of deterioration. Dr. Carrel kept a chicken heart alive for twenty-nine years, and it seemed it would go on forever as long as he continued to do those two things. When he failed to wash away tissue excretions in a timely manner, he would notice that the cells had lower vitality and deterioration. The heart finally died when a co-worker failed to clean away the excretions.

Our bodies work in the same way at the cellular level. If we don't keep our internal systems clean in a timely and regular manner, our vitality level decreases and we become weaker and eventually die.

We cleanse our bodies through a process called *detoxification*. Through herbal formulas, colonics, enemas, fasting, and other methods, we rid the body of excess waste. Once the body starts to eliminate long-stored waste, detoxification begins. In my opinion, the more often we cleanse ourselves internally, the better chance we have of preventing the common diseases that so many suffer from today. Whenever you reflect on health, remember that, although nutrition is important, it's cleansing that makes the difference.

Most people focus on cleansing the outer surfaces of their bodies just about every day. We do this not only so that we look good, but to also feel fresh and clean. Most everyone understands the connection between being clean and being healthy. If only people would devote as much attention to cleansing their insides as they give to their outsides, the steadily increasing disease rates would surely decrease.

When I used to ride the subway in New York City every day, I would notice a brand new subway station with new tracks, looking very clean. Then I would go to the next stop and see old tracks, a dirty station infested with mice and rats. Why didn't these rodents move to the new tracks? Because they are attracted to dirt, and the new tracks were clean. If all the tracks were as clean as those in that new station, not only would the rats not want to visit there, they wouldn't be able to survive. It works the same way in our bodies. Although it's unlikely we'll attract rats, chances are that most of us have infestations of another kind. But if our bodies are clean, these critters won't be able to survive.

There are more than a hundred species of parasites that can live in the human body, causing all sorts of serious problems—from malnutrition to the more advanced stages of disease. Parasites can live anywhere in the body—the lungs, liver, lymph glands, heart, prostate, bile ducts, skin, appendix, muscles, and brain. But most find their homes in the intestinal tract, where they thrive on undigested proteins and processed foods that contribute toward a filthy internal environment. For this reason, cleansing the colon is important. A good colonic series, along with a high-quality herbal program, followed by another colonic or enema, can quickly clean up a toxic environment that took years to produce.

There are other benefits to keeping the colon clean. A clean colon improves the absorption of nutrients, increases peristaltic action of the intestines, which keeps waste moving through smoothly, and improves the flow of the body's energy. I've met people all over the world who have experienced rapid healing and relief from a clean colon.

## The Detox Process

In addition to colon cleansing, cleaning your body internally—at the cellular level—requires not only detoxifying but also fasting. Fasting—refraining from eating solid food—is particularly cleansing because it helps the body release toxic gases that otherwise would find their way into cells. There are numerous ways to expel toxins. The best ways include water fasting, juice fasting, and a cleansing diet.

Detoxification cleans out the great quantity of stored, harmful substances that your body has accumulated over years of eating unhealthful food and being exposed to harmful substances. Detoxification allows the body to do its job and assists it in its cleansing. There are ways to control how quickly you detoxify, and it's very important to go at your own pace. Each person is in a different state of toxicity, so the rate of cleansing should be determined by how you feel.

Detoxifying can make you feel, well, sick, but don't confuse detoxification with actually being diseased or ill. Detoxifying is not always a comfortable process. And it's no wonder: Years of stored toxics are finally leaving the body. Getting clean again won't happen overnight. Some people won't notice any changes during cleansing, but usually the signs are very clear.

The first sign that a detox is working is usually felt above the neck. You may feel like you're coming down with a head cold, or you may get a headache or even a toothache or an ear or eye infection. Many times a rash will develop somewhere on the body. These symptoms may be caused by waste escaping from the body, and there is nothing to be alarmed about unless there is an issue with the heart. During detoxification, the heartbeat may speed up as it pumps more blood to areas that need it, which is normal, but chest pains are an indication that something is seriously wrong and you should seek medical attention.

In extreme cases, the body may detoxify too quickly. If you find you are too sick to stand, or you are in pain, slow down the fast. If you can't feel anything specifically wrong, but you just know something is wrong, it could be a sign that you've detoxified too fast and have exhausted your energy. Remember the formula: if you use too much power and don't have enough energy, you could be doing more harm than good because you've released too much obstruction and your body cannot eliminate it all at once.

Detoxification scares many people, but that's usually only because they don't fully understand it. Health writer Hereward Carrington once said, "Energy is always noted in its expenditure, never in its accumulation. Whenever one feels stronger, he is often getting weaker, because he's expending his strength more rapidly. On the contrary, when feeling weakest, strength is often accumulating most rapidly. It is accumulating and hence unnoticed." You just have to remember that you will probably feel worse before you feel better.

# How To Detox

You can slow down the speed of detoxification by changing your method. The following list presents a guide to a fasting or following a cleansing diet for detoxification. The quickest way to detoxify is to use the suggestion at #5 (water fasting). The next quickest method is #4 (juice fasting), followed by #3 (blended foods), and so on. Let's say you've decided to select the quickest detox method—#5, water fasting—but you begin to have symptoms and need to slow things down. You would immediately go to #4, juice fasting. In another scenario, let's say it's your first detox, and you want to start slowly; perhaps you would start at #2, mono diet, or #3, blended foods.

## Table 1: Fasting or Eating for Detoxification

| INCLUDE | AVOID |
|---|---|
| +5 water fasting | -1 steamed foods |
| +4 juice fasting | -2 grilled foods |
| +3 blended foods | -3 baked foods |
| +2 raw mono diet | -4 processed and packaged foods |
| +1 raw diet with correct food combining | (bread, cereal, etc.) |
| +0 raw diet with incorrect food combining | -5 fried and microwaved foods |

Eating solid food will stop a fast in its tracks; however, when starting to eat after a fast, add food slowly, and don't eat normal-size portions. There are some foods that don't allow cleansing at all and should not be included in your diet; these are indicated on the chart by the negative numbers.

The quickest way to cleanse is to eat nothing, consume only water, and rest. This is known as a water fast, and it will bring about the quickest cleanse and most powerful detoxification. It lets the body do its cleansing work without having to deal with new waste coming in. Remaining work without having to deal with new waste coming in. Remaining active during a water fast is not a good idea, since you need nutrients to stay active; resting will help prevent that loss.

Do not fast on water for more than three days without a trained professional to assist and supervise you. Completely suspend all activities and just stay in bed. Try to have your eyes closed most of the day. A water fast is very cleansing, and one needs to conserve as much energy as possible while on it. If you are water fasting and feel it's too hard on your body, you can slow down the fast and go to a juice fast.

A juice diet is a little easier on the body. It is still very cleansing but not as harsh and brief as a water fast. Even though you should try to be inactive on a juice diet, the same as with a water diet, on a juice diet you're giving the body some calories, so you can be somewhat more active if you choose. Use only freshly made juices. Supermarket juices, including those that are packaged, bottled, or frozen, are usually pasteurized, meaning they've been "cooked" and they're not fresh. The best way to get fresh juice is to make it yourself.

It's best to drink mostly green juices—from leafy green vegetables—with a little carrot or apple mixed in. I don't suggest too much fruit juice; it's usually too sweet and will make you crave sugar. Also, too much sugar pouring into the system too quickly, especially without the fiber from the fruit, may be harmful or could exacerbate a disease. If you do drink fruit juice, always dilute it with a lot of water. The best fruit juice I've found to use on a juice diet is fresh, organic, strained watermelon juice.

The easiest way to conduct a juice fast is to simply replace your standard meals with juice. If you're used to three meals a day, drink a juice at every "mealtime," for a total of three "meals" a day. However, most people eat more than three times a day, so if that applies to you, you may need a little more juice to be satisfied. It's possible to drink too much juice, although drinking fresh juices instead of eating a lot of food is a step in the right direction for health. Eventually, though, you should try to be satisfied with three servings of juice a day.

If a juice diet proves to be too hard on your body, you could add homemade nut milk, such as almond milk, to slow down the cleanse.

The next best way to go on a cleansing diet, or to slow down the cleanse even more, would be to go on a diet of blended foods. The difference between blended foods and juices is that blended foods still retain the fiber along with the juice. With juices, the fiber is removed. Juices are usually considered more cleansing because the body doesn't have to deal with the fiber.

Blended foods are excellent, and I like to make them often. The late Ann Wigmore, founder of the Hippocrates Health Institute and the Ann Wigmore Institute, and a pioneer in the field of raw food nutrition, ate 80 percent of her diet as blended foods. Another name for a blended food is a smoothie, the popular fruit drink. But you can also make vegetable smoothies, often referred to as raw soups and blended salads. (See page 119 through 122.)

To slow detoxification even more, eat a mono diet. A mono diet consists of whole raw food; it slows down cleansing because the body has to do more work to break down the food. Eating mono meals means eating one type of whole food at a time. For example, a meal of only apples is more cleansing than a fruit salad containing many different fruits, because the body has only one type of food to deal with at a time.

To further reduce the detoxification, eat a raw diet, observing the principles of proper food combining. The food-combining chart on page 60 explains the benefits of proper food combining. Once again, the body will have less work to do when we eat foods in proper combinations.

Next, we have a raw food diet that is not properly combined. This consists of high-quality raw food eaten in any order. Usually, raw food recipes—foods with several different ingredients—are in this category.

Although it's not as effective as the other levels of detoxification, it's still cleansing to the body because of the enzymes in raw food. Many people who are just beginning a raw food diet eat combined foods mostly, which are in this category.

When cleansing, we don't need to achieve perfection; by going at our own pace, we can make great strides forward. Anyone switching to a raw food diet would do well eating a good amount of raw food recipes for the first few years. It's not ideal, but it's much better than eating poorly combined cooked foods. Remember, however, that your eating practices should change and progress in accordance with the newly cleansed state of your body. As you begin to eat more healthfully, your body will get cleaner and become more sensitive to harmful foods.

For example, at the outset of a raw food diet, 80 percent of your diet might consist of raw food recipes and only 20 percent of the more cleansing foods. After four or five years of eating this way, it's time to become more disciplined. Your body will be cleaner, and your eating practices should change to go with it. This usually means reversing the earlier stage and consuming 80 to 90 percent of the more cleansing foods and only 10 to 20 percent of the heavier raw food recipes.

During cleansing, cellular rebuilding occurs automatically, although from a dietary standpoint, there are certain foods we can eat to help our bodies rebuild. Usually those foods have the nutrients we're lacking, and these will be different for everyone. Nevertheless, there are numerous foods that are universally advantageous for cleansing—those containing the most liquid.

I believe that dehydration—insufficient water—is a considerable basis for disease today, which is often caused by consuming too many harmful foods in their most damaging forms. The best way to avoid dehydration is to eat moisture-rich foods, which will keep your body clean and free of excess mucus and slime. The more water you drink, the cleaner you should be. If water is your "soap," then you'll want to drink a lot of it to stay clean and free of debris. Water will also help remove the dirt that has been there for so long, causing disease or discomfort.

In many cases, there will be clear signs when something is wrong with your body, and you'll know it's time to detoxify. Other times, it won't be as easy to detect, and you'll have to pay very close attention to your body and its functions. Learn what is supposed to be happening and how your body functions optimally. If it's not functioning at its peak, take it as a sign that something is wrong, whether you feel ill or not. Monitor your digestion, energy, sleeping patterns, and emotions.

A good way to identify a problem is to pay close attention to your digestion. If you're eating three meals a day, you should be going to the bathroom at least twice a day, or at least having one large bowel movement daily. Anything less would signal constipation, which a sure sign your body is not in perfect working order and something needs to change.

## Step Three: Create a Personalized Diet and Lifestyle

We know that the best diet for regaining and maintaining health is raw, ripe, fresh, and organic fruits, vegetables, nuts, and seeds. We also know there is no single eating plan that is best for everyone. Because there are countless variables that determine health, each person's specific dietary needs will differ. For example, someone living in a warmer climate will need to eat more foods with a high water content compared to someone living in a colder climate, where denser foods are necessary. An athlete will need different amounts of nutrients than a more sedentary office worker. We must also take into account each individual's starting point. Someone who has been eating hamburgers and french fries all his life will require a different approach than a vegan who has been eating whole food for many years.

One way to find out your nutrient levels is to have your blood tested. Understanding your blood chemistry is important, because one small oversight can mean the difference between sickness and health. Don't be misled to think you can simply switch to eating a raw food diet overnight and get good results. Success lies in doing the necessary research and understanding what will work best for your own individual chemistry and lifestyle. That is what Step 3 is all about.

Testing the blood to detect deficiencies in any nutrient can tell us exactly what's missing from our diets. But even this can be tricky, because, for example, if you are deficient in calcium, it doesn't necessarily mean you're not getting enough of it from food; it could mean you're consuming too many acid-forming foods or too much protein, or it could point to serious disease. Too much calcium could mean other conditions.

Be sure to seek the help of a professional who understands blood chemistry and can explain the results of your tests. Just because your blood test shows you're lacking a nutrient doesn't automatically mean you should start a regimen of supplements. Seek professional guidance. Then you will know which foods you should eat or avoid to build up your nutrient levels.

## pH

In addition to determining the nutrient levels in our blood, we also need to consider our blood pH when we put together a personalized eating plan. Blood needs to be kept within a certain pH range. If we eat too many acid-forming foods, we could be setting up an environment that is ripe for disease. Eating according to the Formula for Health can ensure that we eat the right balance of acid/alkaline foods.

The acidity of the blood must be kept within a very narrow pH range—mildly basic, or alkaline, at about 7.4, in order to help ward off disease and deficiencies. The pH level of our internal fluids affects every cell in our body, and the entire metabolic process depends on an alkaline environment. The body knows this and will always do its best to ensure the constancy of a correct pH of around 7.4. Just as our body temperature must be maintained at 98.6 degrees F., our blood is ideally maintained at 7.365 pH. No matter how poorly we eat, the body will do whatever it must to make sure the temperature and blood are at their ideal levels.

When the body is acidic, it is vulnerable to germs. The body will work hard to get rid of excessive amounts of acid and will look for more alkalizing minerals. To give our bodies what they need, our diets should be comprised of 80 percent alkaline foods and 20 percent acid foods to maintain the proper pH balance. If the diet drives the blood pH to less alkalizing or more acidic levels than 7.4, we'll run into health problems. Remember the Formula for Health: if the body uses energy trying to maintain its pH balance, it has less energy for other processes. A common sign that we are consuming too many acidic foods is sickness: pain, infection, fatigue, and body malfunctions, including adrenal/thyroid failure, hyperactivity, antisocial behavior, asthma, hemorrhoids, colds and flu, respiratory problems, endometriosis, dry skin and itching, receding gums, finger or toenail fungus, dizziness, joint pain, bad breath, ulcers, colitis, and heartburn.

Today, nearly everyone consumes far too many acidic foods. To balance the blood pH, the body then has to draw out alkalizing minerals, such as magnesium, from other parts of the body (usually the bones) to bring back the balance. The body will literally destroy tissues or systems to regulate its pH priority.

Testing the blood is not the best way to find out your pH balance, because the blood will almost always balance to exactly where it should be. If it didn't, we'd be in the hospital or cemetery. Some people test their urine and saliva with pH strips, but these are not 100 percent accurate

# ALKALINE FOODS

ALKALIZING
VEGETABLES

Alfalfa
Barley grass
Beet greens
Beets
Broccoli
Cabbage
Carrot
Cauliflower
Celery
Chard greens
Chlorella
Collard greens
Cucumber
Dandelions
Dulce
Edible flowers
Eggplant
Fermented veggies
Garlic
Green beans
Green peas
Kale
Kohlrabi
Lettuce
Mushrooms
Mustard greens
Nightshade veggies
Onions
Parsnips (high
  glycemic)
Peas
Peppers
Pumpkin

Radishes
Rutabaga
Sea veggies
Spinach, green
Spirulina
Sprouts
Sweet potatoes
Tomatoes
Watercress
Wheat grass
Wild greens

ALKALIZING
ORIENTAL
VEGETABLES

Daikon
Dandelion root
Kombu
Maitake
Nori
Reishi
Shitake
Umeboshi
Wakame

ALKALIZING FRUITS

Apple
Apricot
Avocado
Banana (high
  glycemic)
Berries
Blackberries
Cantaloupe
Cherries, sour
Coconut, fresh

Currants
Dates, dried
Figs, dried
Grapes
Grapefruit
Honeydew melon
Lemon
Lime
Muskmelons
Nectarine
Orange
Peach
Pear
Pineapple
Raisins
Raspberries
Rhubarb
Strawberries
Tangerine
Tomato
Tropical fruits
Umeboshi plums
Watermelon

ALKALIZING
PROTEIN

Almonds
Chestnuts
Millet
Tempeh (fermented)
Tofu (fermented)
Whey Protein Powder

ALKALIZING
SWEETENERS

Stevia

ALKALIZING
SPICES &
SEASONINGS

Chili pepper
Cinnamon
Curry
Ginger
Herbs (all)
Miso
Mustard
Sea salt
Tamari

ALKALIZING OTHER

Alkaline antioxidant
Water
Apple cider vinegar
Bee pollen
Fresh fruit juice
Green juices
Lecithin granules
Mineral water
Molasses, blackstrap
Probiotic cultures
Soured dairy
Products
Veggie juices

ALKALIZING
MINERALS

Calcium: pH 12
Cesium: pH 14
Magnesium: pH 9
Potassium: pH 14
Sodium: pH 14

Although it might seem that citrus fruits would have an acidifying effect on the body, the citric acid they contain actually has an alkalinizing effect in the system.

Note that a food's acid or alkaline forming tendency in the body has nothing to do with the actual pH of the food itself. For example, lemons are very acidic, however the end products they produce after digestion and assimilation are very alkaline so, lemons are alkaline forming in the body. Likewise, meat will test alkaline before digestion, but it leaves very acidic residue in the body so, like nearly all animal products, meat is very acid forming.

# ACIDIC FOODS

## ACIDIFYING VEGETABLES

Corn
Lentils
Olives
Winter squash

## ACIDIFYING FRUITS

Blueberries
Canned or glazed
  fruits
Cranberries
Currants
Plums**
Prunes**

## ACIDIFYING GRAINS, GRAIN PRODUCTS

Amaranth
Barley
Bran, oat
Bran, wheat
Bread
Corn
Cornstarch
Crackers, soda
Flour, wheat
Flour, white
Hemp seed flour
Kamut
Macaroni
Noodles
Oatmeal
Oats (rolled)
Quinoa
Rice (all)
Rice cakes
Rye
Spaghetti

Spelt
Wheat germ
Wheat

## ACIDIFYING BEANS & LEGUMES

Almond milk
Black beans
Chick peas
Green peas
Kidney beans
Lentils
Pinto beans
Red beans
Rice milk
Soy beans
Soymilk
White beans

## ACIDIFYING DAIRY

Butter
Cheese
Cheese, processed
Ice cream
Ice milk

## ACIDIFYING NUTS & BUTTERS

Cashews
Legumes
Peanut butter
Peanuts
Pecans
Tahini
Walnuts

## ACIDIFYING ANIMAL PROTEIN

Bacon
Beef

Carp
Clams
Cod
Corned beef
Fish
Haddock
Lamb
Lobster
Mussels
Organ meats
Oyster
Pike
Pork
Rabbit
Salmon
Sardines
Sausage
Scallops
Shellfish
Shrimp
Tuna
Turkey
Veal
Venison

## ACIDIFYING FATS & OILS

Avocado oil
Butter
Canola oil
Corn oil
Flax oil
Hemp seed oil
Lard
Olive oil
Safflower oil
Sesame oil
Sunflower oil

## ACIDIFYING SWEETENERS

Carob
Corn syrup
Sugar

## ACIDIFYING ALCOHOL

Beer
Hard liquor
Spirits
Wine

## ACIDIFYING OTHER FOODS

Catsup
Cocoa
Coffee
Mustard
Pepper
Soft drinks
Vinegar

## ACIDIFYING DRUGS & CHEMICALS

Aspirin
Chemicals
Drugs, medicinal
Drugs, psychedelic
Herbicides
Pesticides
Tobacco

## ACIDIFYING JUNK FOOD

Beer: pH 2.5
Coca-Cola: pH 2
Coffee: pH 4

** These foods leave an alkaline ash but have an acidifying effect on the body.

either, because they only measure the levels based on the foods we ate most recently. The only solution is to follow the formula for health and consume the highest-quality foods while avoiding the harmful ones. It's interesting to note that the most harmful and lowest-quality foods are mostly acid forming, and the highest-quality and most health-promoting foods are generally alkalizing.

## Getting It All

The first place to obtain nutrients should be food. If you think you are eating the best possible alkalizing diet and still become nutrient deficient, it could be due to poor absorption caused by prior damage to your system. Another factor could be the quality of today's food. Even nutritious food is not what it once was, because the soil is not as rich in minerals as it used to be. Also, it's not so easy to be able to eat foods at their freshest. · Many nutrients are lost between the time food is picked and the time it is eaten. If we're not getting what we need from food, we need to consider using supplements that contain the missing nutrients.

The best supplements are made from whole food, called "green food" or "superfood." They are generally available as powder, capsules, and pills. These green powders usually contain many nutrients, including chlorophyll, that are commonly missing from the diet. Some of the powders are comprised of carrots, berries, and/or beets, or more uncommon foods, but look for ones that contain a good amount of chlorophyll-rich greens.

If these don't have what you need, I would recommend vitamin and mineral supplements; however, I don't suggest supplements other than enzymes, probiotics, cell food, and green powder until you've had your blood analyzed to see exactly which nutrients are missing.

Even though supplements can play an important role in overcoming your health challenges, do your best to achieve health without relying on them. Supplements are fine for a while. But there is a difference between taking them for a limited time to increase the amount of a particular nutrient you might not be able to get from food and relying on them for the rest of your life. Take supplements if you must, but always look for a better answer—in food.

It is important to understand that a supplement is not a stimulant. Just because a substance gives you a burst of energy doesn't mean it's healthful. There are many companies that sell products that aren't as healthful as they would have you think.

Blood carries nutrients to all parts of the body; it also carries oxygen. In my opinion, every illness—from candida to cancer—is caused by oxygen-deficient, dirty blood. According to the Formula for Health, we need to keep our body as clean as possible. One way is to keep the blood clean and fully oxygenated. If you learn your blood is deficient in oxygen, there are several things you can do to bring that level back up.

Eat high-quality foods, particularly ones that are high in chlorophyll, such as leafy green vegetables, wheatgrass, algae, sea vegetables, and sprouts. Chlorophyll is the pigment that gives trees, grasses, and leafy plants their characteristic green color. More importantly, chlorophyll enables plants to convert the sun's energy into nutrients that can be utilized by other living organisms. Chlorophyll is similar to the hemoglobin in human blood. Chlorophyll-rich plant juices supply an abundance of minerals, vitamins, and proteins, plus they contain oxygen.

## Step Four: Emotional and Spiritual Growth

To put the Formula for Health into action, you will need to include more than just dietary changes; you will need emotional support and mental grounding, both of which begin with knowledge. Knowledge will give you the foundation to proceed. Forget what you think you know about health and find the truth that will support health. Don't settle for what you want to hear.

When you learn the correct information, make sure you understand it completely, because knowledge without understanding is virtually useless. Once you have knowledge and understanding, you will have wisdom:

## Knowledge + Understanding = Wisdom

With wisdom, it's easy to then put your plan into action. So many health seekers fail at achieving their goals because they lack the wisdom to get through the hard times. Wisdom helps establish your correct pace so you don't go too fast. My advice is to not go beyond your understanding of health. If you get ahead of yourself or your understanding, you're going to set yourself up for failure.

How can you know what your optimal pace is? It's very simple: if you're not seeing results, you're going too slowly, and if you're not enjoying the changes, you're going too fast. When you begin this diet with an awareness of why you're on it, you should keep at the right pace. Only those who rush into something before they know why they're doing it or how to do it will run into problems. Let's face it—we will all have moments of struggle in changing our way of eating and living due to our health challenges. But wisdom will keep us strong and carry us past those moments.

Once your plan is in action and you see that it's working, you will feel joy; then it all becomes easier. It might take a little time to get there— some people will take longer than others—but once you do, that's when life becomes fun. Amazingly, you can use this information not just for diet and health. You can apply it to every aspect of your life. If you have wisdom, you will have joy, and it's joy that will give you the two keys to success at anything in life: efficiency and consistency.

How you do anything is how you do everything. Efficiency is wisdom in motion. The key to wisdom is to be so efficient that you can get the most results out of the least work. So many people today are extremely inefficient; they do the most work and end up getting the least results. We need to turn that around. When everything is going the right way and at the right pace, we can stop looking for answers and start enjoying life.

So many people fail today because they're never satisfied; they're always looking for new ways to do things. They go back and forth too much. Having an open mind is so important, and there is nothing wrong with trying new things to see if they'll work. But you must give what you're already doing a chance. You have to do something consistently to see if it will give you the results you desire. If you jump from thing to thing, you will not come up with the answers you're looking for. Efficiency will lead to consistency.

## Efficiency + Consistency = Confidence

Confidence is the groundwork for enthusiasm. When it comes to overcoming your shortfalls and thriving, enthusiasm makes the difference. Remember that confidence does not mean pride. Confidence means you have a well-grounded understanding and the patience to wait for the answers, but also a willingness to admit when you are wrong. All of this leads to more knowledge.

If you're not happy with your results, you must change their cause. If you keep doing the same things, you will continue to create the same outcomes. You must change what you're doing to get new results.

Building a personal relationship with our Creator has helped me overcome my addictions and enjoy emotional peace. Consistent prayer enables me to find the answers I need to keep going forward. For more information about building health through spirituality, please read my book *Health According to the Scriptures* (343 Publishing Company, 2007).

---

## Sugar Dangers

"In my opinion, the number one type of food that deranges the biological terrain is any food that is high in sugar. This sugar is not limited to white sugar but includes fruits that contain a high amount of sugar or have a high-glycemic index. Microforms love all forms of sugar, especially those that cause a rapid rise of blood sugar (cane sugars and corn sugars). The more sugar harmful microforms get, the faster they will reproduce, and the faster they reproduce, the more they are decomposing and fermenting your body from the inside." —Gabriel Cousens, MD

---

# Chapter 6

# Putting a Plan Together

Now that you have all this information, what do you do with it? How do you go about implementing it all?

I have formulated a model plan to help you make a successful transition to a healthier lifestyle, taking into consideration all that I've talked about up to this point. I realize, however, that every person is different, so as you read my plan, keep in mind that you can make adjustments depending on your particular limitations, work schedule, and other factors. For example, a person with children will not have as much time and freedom as a single person. Someone who works nights obviously can't go to sleep at the same time as someone with a day job. These are my suggestions based on the ideal, and I only ask that you do your best. You don't have to follow the plan 100 percent to reap major benefits.

First, let's recap the best of the best (and worst of the worst). Always keep these in mind and try to hit these goals as you strive for health:

- Best-quality foods: fruits, vegetables, nuts, and seeds that are raw, ripe, fresh, and organic
- Best form in which to consume foods: liquefied—juiced, blended, or thoroughly chewed
- Best way to consume foods: proper food combining or sequential eating (see pages 55 to 60)
- Best quantity of food: just the amount that satisfies our needs
- Best foods to consume: alkaline, chlorophyll-rich foods, such as leafy green vegetables, wheatgrass, and sprouts
- Foods to avoid: acid-forming, processed foods, such as any packaged or canned food, grains, flour and flour-containing products
- Worst ways to prepare food: frying and microwaving

# Three Levels To Success

The best way to make a simple and easy transition to a higher-quality diet is to be consistent, continue to gain knowledge about the top foods for your health, and enjoy the experience of tasting new foods. Once you detoxify, you can transition from level to level until you reach the point that is best for you. There are three levels to a successful diet: the Cleansing Diet, the Transition Diet, and the Maintenance Diet. (Please read chapter 5 before embarking on these diets, and refer to it regularly while you are making your transition.)

## The Cleansing Diet

The less you eat, the faster your body will clean out, and that is the basis for the Cleansing Diet, a liquid detoxification diet that can include any or all of the following: water fasting, juice fasting, and blending. There are supplementary practices that can be done in addition to these food recommendations, such as herbal cleanses, enemas, colonics, and other cleansing treatments, but for the purposes of this book, I'm focusing only on the food aspects. I suggest reading further on these other topics if you are interested in them. Adding these treatments to the Cleansing Diet will enhance any cleanse and give you the best results.

The quickest way to cleanse is not to eat at all: to go on a water or juice fast. I've known people who fast for a few days, and others who can fast for a few weeks at a time. Unless you can stay in bed for three days, I don't recommend a water fast; it can be difficult for the first-timer. When you're just starting out, I recommend a three-day juice fast, which means drinking only green vegetable juices. Fruit juices are too high in sugar; leave those for the next stage.

In the future, after you've successfully managed a raw food diet, you can go on a Cleansing Diet anytime, for shorter or longer periods, whenever you feel the need. The optimum method for keeping your body clean once you're on the Maintenance Diet is to fast one day each week.

## The Transition Diet

The Transition Diet is an introduction to a raw food diet. Between the transitional stage and the Maintenance Diet, just about any raw, ripe, fresh, and organic fruit or vegetable is fine in any amount. Although this is not ideal—for example, overeating raw organic dates is not advised because of their sugar content—it's far less harmful than any of the sugary, processed, or animal-based foods you may have eaten in the past or are still eating now. Eventually, as you get healthier, you'll want to refine your diet, not only focusing on the quality of your food, but also on the quantity.

During the Transition Diet, you will begin to heed the principles of food combining (see chapter 4) and focus mostly on leafy green vegetables. If you have been used to eating the standard American diet, this is the stage where you avoid or at least cut way back on animal products, processed food, fat, and sugar. At least 75 percent of your Transition Diet should be raw, ripe, fresh, organic fruits, vegetables, nuts, and seeds.

During the Transition Diet, slight symptoms of discomfort may appear as part of the cleansing process, similar to those you may have experienced on the Cleansing Diet. People who don't understand how the body works might take these symptoms as negative signs—the reason it's so vital to understand the relationship between health and nutrition before getting ahead of yourself. The most common reason people. give up during the Transition Diet is because they don't understand that these symptoms are a natural part of cleansing as a result of eating this healthful way; these symptoms will clear up as they get healthier.

However, if a Transition Diet is done at a moderate pace—that is, if a person gradually incorporates more healthful foods while gradually adapting food-combining principles and eliminating harmful foods—there should be few uncomfortable symptoms.

If you're faced with a specific health challenge, you may have to go to the Maintenance Diet sooner. If not, you may stay on the Transition Diet as long as two years, when it's best to then move on to the Maintenance Diet. Once the body is clean, once our chemistry improves, the diet needs to change as well. The cleaner we become, the better our diet has to become.

## The Maintenance Diet

Although you may go back and forth among the diets over the years, it's important to get to a point where you are following the Maintenance Diet the most. More than the other two diets, the Maintenance Diet is individually tailored and geared to your lifestyle. At this level, you will focus solely on raw, ripe, fresh, organic fruits, vegetables, nuts, and seeds. Foods should come from the best sources available, and you will adhere to the food-combining principles at all times. You will avoid most animal foods, processed foods, processed sugar, and cooked fats.

## Do Your Best

This all may seem daunting, but I always advise people to do the best they can. As the years go by, you'll continue to fine-tune your diet; you'll find more sources for fresher, riper foods, learn more recipes for blending and juicing, experiment with combinations, and discover just how much or how little food your body really needs to be healthy. Your body will let you know when you need a cleanse and what type of cleanse you need. You'll learn instinctively how to keep your body supplied with the nutrients it needs, while conserving as much energy as possible.

Technically, the Cleansing Diet and the Transition Diet both cleanse the system. But if you feel like you can't or don't want to detox on the Cleansing Diet, that's fine; do not rush into things you're not sure of. The

Transition Diet will also cleanse your system; it will just take a little longer. As long as you go at a steady, comfortable pace, you should avoid any possible issues that may come up with cleansing too quickly. You will still benefit, because once you've eliminated harmful foods, your body will be stronger than when you started. You can always go back to the Cleansing Diet to help rid yourself of the toxins that have built up in your system. After your body cleans out, though, remember to eat only healthful foods so the toxins don't return.

# The Important Foods

Take time to learn as much as you can about food. Fruits and vegetables are available everywhere and their variety is amazing. There are more than just apples and bananas and green beans to experience. Many are available in local markets that we pass every day. Include as many as you can in your daily diet so you don't get bored. The following lists include the foods you should emphasize in your formula for health.

## Fresh Vegetables

Most of your daily diet should come from fresh vegetables.
- **Salad greens.** Our diet should be primarily made up of fresh, chlorophyll-rich, leafy greens. You'll find many in your market or natural food store that you may have never heard of before. Try new ones as often as possible. Here are some of the more common ones: arugula, bok choy, chicory, collard greens, dandelion, garlic greens, kale, lettuce (many varieties), mustard greens, spinach, Swiss chard, turnip greens, watercress, and sunflower greens.
- **Other vegetables.** These vegetables are good choices: asparagus, broccoli, cabbage, cauliflower, celery, and green beans. Carrots, corn, parsnips, and white potatoes are high in carbohydrates and should be eaten very sparingly.

## Fresh Fruits

Any plant containing a seed or seeds is technically a fruit. The more liquid a fruit has, the better it is for you. Other than melons, fruits that are commonly considered to be vegetables (such as tomatoes) usually have the most liquid and are the most healthful.

The following sweet fruits should be limited or eaten in small amounts: apples, avocados, bell peppers, berries, cantaloupes, cherries, cucumbers, grapes, grapefruits, kiwifruit, lemons, melons, papayas, pears, persimmons, pineapples, squash, and zucchini.

Make certain the fruit you eat is fully ripe, not hard. Fruits that are commonly picked unripe include bananas, mangoes, oranges, peaches, pineapples, and plums.

## Nuts and Seeds

Nuts and seeds are best eaten after they have been soaked for six to twelve hours, because soaking releases enzymes that allow for easier digestion. It's very easy to eat too many nuts, so be careful. Try not to eat more than one cup of nuts a day. For nuts, choose almonds, filberts, pecans, walnuts, and young coconuts. For seeds, choose flax, hemp, pumpkin, sesame, and sunflower.

## Whole Grains

It's best to eat grains that have been sprouted first, as they are easier to digest. The most healthful grains are amaranth, buckwheat (hulled), millet, quinoa, and teff. The least healthful grains are barley, corn, rice (white and white basmati), rye, spelt, and wheat.

## Sea Vegetables

There are many different types of sea vegetables. Here are a few of the most popular with their most important benefits:

**Alaria.** Delicious raw in salads, either presoaked or marinated, alaria is comparable to whole sesame seeds in their calcium content (1100mg/100g). It also has a very high vitamin A content, comparable to parsley, spinach, or turnip greens, and is very high in B vitamins.

**Arame.** Arame has a nutty taste and is high in calcium, phosphorous, iodine, iron, potassium, and vitamins A and B.

**Dulse.** Delicious as a raw snack, dulse has a distinctive, strong sea flavor. It is also great in salads and contains about 22 percent protein, which is more than almonds, chickpeas, and whole sesame seeds. A handful of dulse provides a whole day's supply of iron and fluoride. The same handful will provide more than 100 percent of the RDA for vitamin B6 and 66 percent of the RDA for vitamin $B_{12}$. Dulse is relatively low in sodium (1740mg/100g) and high in potassium (7820mg/100g). Dulse is also an excellent source of naturally occurring manganese, fluoride, copper, and zinc.

**Hijiki.** Hijiki is very high in calcium, vitamins A, $B_1$, and $B_2$, and phosphorous.

**Kelp.** Kelp tastes great marinated. It is exceptionally high in all the major minerals, particularly calcium, potassium, magnesium, and iron. It is also rich in important trace minerals, such as manganese, copper, and zinc. One ounce of kelp provides the recommended daily dose of chromium, which is instrumental in blood sugar regulation. That same ounce provides many times the RDA for iodine, which is essential to the thyroid gland.

**Nori.** Nori has a distinctive, mild, nutty, salty-sweet taste. It is great in salads and can be used to make vegetable sushi rolls. It contains about 28 percent protein, which is more than lentils, sunflower seeds, and wheat germ. Of all the sea vegetables, nori is the highest in vitamins $B_1$, $B_2$, $B_6$, C, and E.

## Fermented Foods

Fermented foods have been inoculated with a "friendly" bacterial culture, such as acidophilus, bifidus, or koji, to name just a few. Examples of fermented foods are amazake, kimchi, miso, sauerkraut, seed cheese, and organic yogurt.

Fermented foods have several health benefits. Important friendly bacteria grow during the fermentation process, and they encourage healthy intestinal flora and regular bowel movements. Thus some fermented foods can be very healthful and healing. However, many people are on nutritious diets that don't include any fermented foods and they are in excellent health.

## Sprouted Food

Sprouted food refers to any type of seed, nut, grain, or bean that has been soaked in water, exposed to air and indirect sunlight, rinsed daily, and has started to form a new plant, beginning with a sprout. Some examples include almond sprouts, buckwheat sprouts, mung bean sprouts, and sunflower sprouts. Sprouted foods are some of the highest quality forms of food you can put into your body. They are very helpful for building new cells and provide the cells with oxygen. Green sprouts are very high in chlorophyll.

## My Journey—and Yours

It has been a long journey for me. As I was growing up, I never even entertained the dream of becoming a health writer and never cared what I ate. As I grew older, I grew wiser. I am so blessed to have found the formula for health.

A good friend of mine is a medical doctor, and I showed him Arnold Ehret's books years ago. He gave me the same response most doctors do. Today, more than eighty years after Ehret's death, the formula still works. There will always be new foods and new dietary ideas and fads, but the formula for health will never change. I'm glad you picked up this book, and now you know the formula too. Simply apply it and you will start to achieve the three blessings we all want:

1. To cure disease  2. To prevent disease  3. To stay looking young

# Chapter 7

# Three-Week Action Meal Plan

To help you put the Formula for Health into action, I've put together a twenty-one-day menu and life planner that will help turn your life around. My favorite recipes can be found in chapter 8, but there are no limits to the wonderfully delicious and different recipes you can enjoy on a raw food diet, so feel free to change, add, and adjust recipes as much as you like.

The first thing you will notice about my plan is that I suggest eating only two meals a day, with no snacking between meals. If you're used to three meals a day, this may take some getting used to, but once you start eating high-quality food and your body has cleaned out, you'll find that a meal's worth of food is enough, and you should not have a desire for food at other times of the day. If you feel this is too much of a change and you need three meals a day, just make sure your last meal is eaten by 7:00 p.m. Do not consume food after 7:00 p.m. Of course, you don't have to be completely rigid about this—sometimes it cannot be helped—but as a general rule, try not to eat too late.

Also, do not drink water with your meals. Drink water one hour before or one hour after your meals, but not with your meals.

Try to get at least eight hours of sleep a night. If you are not able to eat at these times, or if you're not willing to eat your first meal so early, you may adjust the times. For example, instead of eating at 9:00 a.m. and 3:00 p.m., eat at noon and 6:00 p.m. The times listed are ideal, though, so do your best to get in the habit.

And, as I discussed in the previous chapter, as you become more adept at the Transition and Maintenance Diets, try to fast one day a week, taking only water and/or juice. (Make sure all juices are freshly squeezed and diluted 75 percent with water.)

# Suggested Daily Schedule

**6:00 A.M.** Arise.

Upon rising, drink 2 cups of clean water (spring, filtered, ionized, or distilled). If using distilled water, add the juice of 1 lemon to add back the minerals. Now is also the time to exercise.

**7:00 A.M.** Drink 2 cups of green vegetable juice.

Drink 2 cups of green vegetable juice made from 80 percent green leafy vegetables and, if desired, 20 percent sweet vegetables. Here are some suggested juice combinations:

• apple, cabbage, kale
• beet, celery, cucumber, kale
• carrot, cucumber, parsley, spinach
• celery, cucumber, spinach
• watermelon juice (with rind) is acceptable on occasion

**9:00 A.M.** First meal of the day.
Eat sprouted grains with blended raw salad, low-sugar fruit, and your choice of a raw food recipe.

**NOON.** Drink 2 cups of water or green vegetable juice.

**3:00 P.M.** Second meal of the day.
Eat salad with a dressing made from avocado, soaked nuts or seeds (sunflower, pumpkin, or sesame seeds), or a recommended cold-pressed oil with your favorite herbs.

**6:00 P.M.** Drink 2 cups of water or green vegetable juice, if you are hungry.

# Twenty-One Days of Menu Plans

Following are sample meal plans to get you started. The meals do not have to be eaten in order; for example, you can go from Day 2 to Day 19 or skip around as you like. However, all foods should be raw, ripe, fresh, and organic.

**DAY 1:** 7:00 A.M. Juice of 1 cup spinach, 1 cucumber, 2 stalks celery

9:00 A.M. Green apples or berries and a salad, if desired

Noon. Juice of 1 cup kale, 1 cucumber, 1 green apple, 2 cabbage leaves

3:00 P.M. Paul's Powerful Salad (page 105) or Every-Need-Met Salad (page 105) with Tahini Dressing (page 104), Onion-Walnut Pâté (page 108), and Mushroom Pizza (page 109)

6:00 P.M. Juice of 1 cup spinach, 3 stalks celery, 3 carrots

**DAY 2:** 7:00 A.M. Juice of 1 cup spinach, 1 cucumber, 2 stalks celery

9:00 A.M. Fruit of your choice and soaked nuts

NOON. Juice of 1 cup buckwheat greens, 1 carrot, 1 stalk celery, 1 cucumber

3:00 P.M. Mushroom Pizza (page 109) and Paul's Powerful Salad (page 105)

6:00 P.M. Juice of 1 cup sunflower sprouts, 1 cup cabbage, 3 kale leaves, 1 carrot

**DAY 3:** 7:00 A.M. Juice of 1 cup spinach, 1 cucumber, 2 stalks celery

9:00 A.M. Melon (watermelon, honeydew, cantaloupe, etc.)

**Noon.** Juice of 1 stalk celery, 1 cucumber, 1 cup spinach, 3 beet greens, 2 carrots

**3:00 P.M.** Avocado with Salsa (page 108), Cauliflower "Mashed Potatoes" (page 112), and Raw Fudge (page 118)

**6:00 P.M.** Juice of 3 collard green leaves, 2 beets, 1 apple

**DAY 4:** **7:00 A.M.** Juice of 1 cup spinach, 1 cucumber, 2 stalks celery

**9:00 A.M.** Banana "Ice Cream" (page 118) and Raw Fudge (page 118)

**NOON.** Juice of 1 cup greens (any kind), 2 carrots, 1 apple

**3:00 P.M.** Spanish "Rice" (page 110) and Sweet Annie Kale Salad (page 106)

**6:00 P.M.** Juice of 1 cup spinach, 1 cucumber, 1 lemon, 2 kale leaves

**DAY 5:** **7:00 A.M.** Juice of 1 cup spinach, 1 cucumber, 2 stalks celery

**9:00 A.M.** Strawberry "Cheesecake" (page 116) and Nut Milk (page 121)

**NOON.** Juice of 1 cup buckwheat greens, 1 red bell pepper, 1 handful parsley, 1 beet

**3:00 P.M.** Everybody's Favorite Salad (page 106) and Chinese Broccoli with Pine Nuts (page 111)

**6:00 P.M.** Juice of 2 cups parsley, 1 lemon, 2 beets

**DAY 6:** **7:00 A.M.** Juice of 1 cup spinach, 1 cucumber, 2 stalks celery

**9:00 A.M.** Banana "Ice Cream" (page 118) and Raw Fudge (page 118)

**NOON.** Juice of 1 cup spinach, 1 cup watercress, 1-inch cube peeled fresh ginger, 1 apple

**3:00 P.M.** Salad of your choice and Mushroom Pizza (page 109)

**6:00 P.M.** Juice of 1 cup sunflower sprouts, 1 cup cabbage, 3 kale leaves, 1 carrot

**DAY 7:** **7:00 A.M.** Juice of 1 cup spinach, 1 cucumber, 2 stalks celery

**9:00 A.M.** Blended salad of your choice and flax crackers

**NOON.** Juice of 1 cup kale, 1 cucumber, 1 green apple, 2 cabbage leaves.

**3:00 P.M.** Smoothie made with your choice of fruit and greens

**6:00 P.M.** Juice of 1 cup spinach, 3 stalks celery, 3 carrots

**DAY 8:** **7:00 A.M.** Juice of 1 cup spinach, 1 cucumber, 2 stalks celery

**9:00 A.M.** Fruit of your choice and soaked nuts

**NOON.** Juice of 1 cup buckwheat greens, 1 carrot, 1 stalk celery, 1 cucumber

**3:00 P.M.** Mushroom Pizza (page 109) and Paul's Powerful Salad (page 105)

**6:00 P.M.** Juice of 1 cup sunflower sprouts, 1 cup cabbage, 3 kale leaves, 1 carrot

**DAY 9:** **7:00 A.M.** Juice of 1 cup spinach, 1 cucumber, 2 stalks celery

**9:00 A.M.** Green apples or berries and a salad, if desired

**NOON.** Juice of 1 stalk celery, 1 cucumber, 1 cup spinach, 3 beet greens, 2 carrots

**3:00 P.M.** Paul's Powerful Salad (page 105) or Every-Need-Met Salad (page 105) with Tahini Dressing (page 104), Onion-Walnut Pâté (page 108), and Mushroom Pizza (page 109)

**6:00 P.M.** Juice of 3 collard green leaves, 2 beets, 1 apple

# Twenty-One Days of Menu Plans

**DAY 10:** 7:00 A.M. Juice of 1 cup spinach, 1 cucumber, 2 stalks celery

9:00 A.M. Banana "Ice Cream" (page 118) and Raw Fudge (page 118)

NOON. Juice of 1 cup greens of any kind, 2 carrots, 1 apple

3:00 P.M. Spanish "Rice" (page 110) and Sweet Annie Kale Salad (page 106)

6:00 P.M. Juice of 1 cup spinach, 1 cucumber, 1 lemon, 2 kale leaves

**DAY 11:** 7:00 A.M. Juice of 1 cup spinach, 1 cucumber, 2 stalks celery

9:00 A.M. Strawberry "Cheesecake" (page 116) and Nut Milk (page 121)

NOON. Juice of 1 cup buckwheat greens, 1 red bell pepper, 1 cup parsley, 1 beet

3:00 P.M. Everybody's Favorite Salad (page 106) and Chinese Broccoli with Pine Nuts (page 111)

6:00 P.M. Juice of 2 cups parsley, 1 lemon, 2 beets

**DAY 12:** 7:00 A.M. Juice of 1 cup spinach, 1 cucumber, 2 stalks celery

9:00 A.M. Melon (watermelon, honeydew, cantaloupe, etc.)

NOON. Juice of 1 cup spinach, 1 cup watercress, 1-inch cube peeled fresh ginger, 1 apple

3:00 P.M. Avocado with Salsa (page 108), Cauliflower "Mashed Potatoes" (page 112), and Raw Fudge (page 118)

6:00 P.M. Juice of 1 cup sunflower sprouts, 1 cup cabbage, 3 kale leaves, 1 carrot

**DAY 13:** 7:00 A.M. Juice of 1 cup spinach, 1 cucumber, 2 stalks celery

9:00 A.M. Blended salad of your choice with flax crackers

NOON. Juice of 1 cup kale, 1 cucumber, 1 green apple, 2 cabbage leaves

3:00 P.M. Salad of your choice and Mushroom Pizza (page 109)

6:00 P.M. Juice of 1 cup spinach, 3 celery stalks, 3 carrots

**DAY 14:** 7:00 A.M. Juice of 1 cup spinach, 1 cucumber, 2 stalks celery

9:00 A.M. Green apples or berries and a salad, if desired

NOON. Juice of 1 cup buckwheat greens, 1 carrot, 1 stalk celery, 1 cucumber

3:00 P.M. Paul's Powerful Salad (page 105) or Every-Need-Met Salad (page 105) with Tahini Dressing (page 104), Onion-Walnut Pâté (page 108), and Mushroom Pizza (page 109)

6:00 P.M. Juice of 1 cup sunflower sprouts, 1 cup cabbage, 3 kale leaves, 1 carrot

**DAY 15:** 7:00 A.M. Juice of 1 cup spinach, 1 cucumber, 2 stalks celery

9:00 A.M. Blended salad of your choice with flax crackers

NOON. Juice of 1 stalk celery, 1 cucumber, 1 cup spinach, 3 beet greens, 2 carrots

3:00 P.M. Blended salad of your choice with flax crackers

6:00 P.M. Juice of 3 collard green leaves, 2 beets, 1 apple

# Twenty-One Days of Menu Plans

**DAY 16:** 7:00 A.M. Juice of 1 cup spinach, 1 cucumber, 2 stalks celery

9:00 A.M. Smoothie made with your choice of fruit and greens

NOON. Juice of 1 cup greens of any kind, 2 carrots, 1 apple

3:00 P.M. Mushroom Pizza (page 109)

6:00 P.M. Juice of 1 cup spinach, 1 cucumber, 1 lemon, 2 kale leaves

**DAY 17:** 7:00 A.M. Juice of 1 cup spinach, 1 cucumber, 2 stalks celery

9:00 A.M. Blended salad of your choice with flax crackers

NOON. Juice of 1 cup buckwheat greens, 1 red bell pepper, 1 cup parsley, 1 beet

3:00 P.M. Everybody's Favorite Salad (page 106) and Chinese Broccoli with Pine Nuts (page 111)

6:00 P.M. Juice of 2 cups parsley, 1 lemon, 2 beets

**DAY 18:** 7:00 A.M. Juice of 1 cup spinach, 1 cucumber, 2 stalks celery

9:00 A.M. Banana "Ice Cream" (page 118) and Raw Fudge (page 118)

NOON. Juice of 1 cup spinach, 1 cup watercress, 1-inch cube peeled fresh ginger, 1 apple

3:00 P.M. Spanish "Rice" (page 110) and Sweet Annie Kale Salad (page 106)

6:00 P.M. Juice of 1 cup sunflower sprouts, 1 cup cabbage, 3 kale leaves, 1 carrot

**DAY 19:** 7:00 A.M. Juice of 1 cup spinach, 1 cucumber, 2 stalks celery

9:00 A.M. Melon (watermelon, honeydew, cantaloupe, etc.)

NOON. Juice of 1 cup kale, 1 cucumber, 1 green apple, 2 cabbage leaves

3:00 P.M. Avocado with Salsa (page 108), Cauliflower "Mashed Potatoes" (page 112), and Raw Fudge (page 118)

6:00 P.M. Juice of 1 cup spinach, 3 celery stalks, 3 carrots

**DAY 20:** 7:00 A.M. Juice of 1 cup spinach, 1 cucumber, 2 stalks celery

9:00 A.M. Fruit of your choice and soaked nuts

NOON. Juice of 1 cup buckwheat greens, 1 carrot, 1 stalk celery, 1 cucumber

3:00 P.M. Mushroom Pizza (page 109) and Paul's Powerful Salad (page 105)

6:00 P.M. Juice of 1 cup sunflower sprouts, 1 cup cabbage, 3 kale leaves, 1 carrot

**DAY 21:** 7:00 A.M. Juice of 1 cup spinach, 1 cucumber, 2 stalks celery

9:00 A.M. Green apples or berries and salad, if desired

NOON. Juice of 1 stalk celery, 1 cucumber, 1 cup spinach, 3 beet greens, 2 carrots

3:00 P.M. Paul's Powerful Salad (page 105) or Every-Need-Met Salad (page 105) with Tahini Dressing (page 104), Onion-Walnut Pâté (page 108), and Mushroom Pizza (page 109)

6:00 P.M. Juice of 3 collard green leaves, 2 beets, 1 apple

# Chapter 8

# Raw Food Recipes

## TAHINI DRESSING

**YIELD: 5 SERVINGS**

*This is a delicious, all-purpose salad dressing you can use all year long. Store it covered, in the refrigerator. Nama Shoyu is raw, unpasteurized Japanese soy sauce. Look for it in natural food stores or online.*

$1/2$ cup raw tahini

Juice of $1/2$ medium-size lemon

1 clove garlic

Pinch of cayenne

Nama Shoyu

Combine the tahini, lemon juice, garlic, and cayenne in a blender and process until completely smooth. With the blender running, add water, 1 to 2 teaspoons at a time, until the dressing is the consistency you desire. Season with Nama Shoyu to taste.

## TOMATO BASIL DRESSING

**YIELD: 3 SERVINGS**

*This dressing is especially delicious in late summer, when you're assured of fresh, ripe tomatoes and basil.*

2 ripe tomatoes, cut into quarters

1 cup fresh basil leaves

Juice of $1/2$ medium-size lemon

1 clove garlic

Combine all of the ingredients in a blender or food processor and process until completely smooth.

# PAUL'S POWERFUL SALAD

YIELD: 1 SERVING

*I call this salad "powerful" because every ingredient is a powerhouse of nutrients.*

Fresh spinach leaves (as much as you like)
1 ripe avocado, peeled, pitted, and chopped
1/2 medium-size cucumber, chopped
1/2 red bell pepper, cored, seeded, and chopped (optional)
1/2 stalk celery, chopped
Juice of 1 lemon
1 to 2 tablespoons ground flaxseeds

Place the spinach, avocado, cucumber, optional bell pepper, and celery in a large bowl. Toss gently to combine. Sprinkle with the lemon juice and flaxseeds.

# EVERY-NEED-MET SALAD

YIELD: 1 SERVING

*This salad will meet your every need for nutrition.*

1 ripe avocado, peeled, pitted, and chopped
1/2 medium-size cucumber, chopped
1 stalk celery, chopped
1/2 cup dulse, soaked for 30 seconds, then drained and chopped
1/2 red bell pepper, cored, seeded, and chopped (optional)
1 to 2 tablespoons ground flaxseeds

Combine the avocado, cucumber, celery, dulse, and optional bell pepper in a large bowl. Toss gently to combine. Sprinkle with the flaxseeds.

# Sweet Annie Kale Salad

**YIELD: 4 TO 6 SERVINGS**

*Kale is bursting with nutrients, and I love the combination of the sweet and bitter flavors in this salad.*

 1 bunch kale, stemmed and chopped
 $\frac{1}{2}$ cup raisins
 $\frac{1}{4}$ cup cold-pressed extra-virgin olive oil
 $\frac{1}{4}$ cup unpasteurized raw honey
 2 tablespoons pine nuts
 1 clove garlic, minced

Combine all of the ingredients in a large bowl. Massage them with your hands for 5 minutes to soften the kale and blend the flavors.

# Everybody's Favorite Salad

**YIELD: 4 SERVINGS**

*This recipe is a standard part of my repertoire.*

 2 large heads romaine lettuce, chopped
 2 ripe avocados, peeled, pitted, and chopped
 2 ripe tomatoes, diced
 $\frac{1}{4}$ cup pine nuts
 $\frac{1}{4}$ cup raisins
 3 tablespoons cold-pressed extra-virgin olive oil
 1 tablespoon freshly squeezed lemon juice
 2 teaspoons sea salt
 2 teaspoons raw apple cider vinegar
 1 teaspoon crushed red pepper flakes

Combine all of the ingredients in a large bowl. Mix well. Let the salad rest for 10 minutes before serving.

# Raw Healthful Pesto

*Serve as a dip or as a sauce over raw "pasta."*

2 to 4 cloves garlic
2 bunches spinach
1 bunch fresh basil
1 cup pine nuts
$1/2$ cup cold-pressed extra-virgin olive oil
Juice of $1/2$ medium-size lemon
$1/2$ teaspoon sea salt

Place the garlic in a food processor and process until it is well minced. Add all of the remaining ingredients and process until completely smooth.

# Tomato Sauce

YIELD: ABOUT 2 CUPS

*I like to cut up an avocado, mix it in with this sauce, and serve it over raw "pasta."*

3 ripe tomatoes, cut into quarters
$1/2$ cup sun-dried tomatoes (not packed in oil)
1 small hot chile (such as jalapeño or serrano)
$1^1/2$ teaspoons chopped fresh basil
$1^1/2$ teaspoons chopped fresh oregano
1 clove garlic

Place all of the ingredients in a blender or food processor and process until completely smooth.

# Avocado with Salsa

**YIELD: 1 SERVING**

*Once you start making your own salsa, you'll never go back to the jarred stuff.*

  2 ripe plum tomatoes, cut into quarters
  1 tablespoon freshly squeezed lemon juice
  1½ teaspoons minced onion
  1½ teaspoons chopped fresh cilantro
  1 teaspoon cold-pressed extra-virgin olive oil
  ½ teaspoon Nama Shoyu
  ½ clove garlic, chopped
  Pinch of cayenne
  1 ripe avocado, peeled, pitted, and cut in half

Place the tomatoes, lemon juice, onion, cilantro, olive oil, Nama Shoyu, garlic, and cayenne in a food processor and process or pulse just until well combined but still chunky. Pour the salsa into the avocado halves.


# Onion-Walnut Pâté

**YIELD: 5 TO 8 SERVINGS**

*This is great served with raw vegetables, or slice it and serve it as an entrée.*

  2 cups soaked walnuts
  1 cup minced onions
  ¼ cup loosely packed fresh parsley
  2 teaspoons pine nuts
  Sea salt

Place the walnuts, onions, parsley, and pine nuts in a blender and process until completely smooth. Season with sea salt to taste.

# PINE NUT DIP

**YIELD: 2 CUPS**

*Pour this over a raw salad or use it as a dip for raw fresh vegetables.*

1 cup pine nuts
Juice of $\frac{1}{2}$ medium-size lemon
1 (1-inch) cube peeled fresh ginger
1 clove garlic
$\frac{1}{4}$ teaspoon ground nutmeg
Sea salt

Place the pine nuts, lemon juice, ginger, garlic, and nutmeg in a blender or food processor and process until well combined. Season with sea salt to taste.

# MUSHROOM PIZZA

**YIELD: 1 SERVING**

*Who says you can't have a raw pizza?*

1 large portobello mushroom
1 lemon
$\frac{1}{4}$ cup raw tahini or almond butter
1 ripe tomato, thinly sliced
$\frac{1}{4}$ ripe avocado, peeled, pitted, and thinly sliced (optional)

Remove and discard the stem of the mushroom and clean the mushroom cap. Turn the cap upside down and place it on a serving plate. Squeeze the lemon juice over it, then pour on the tahini. Top with the tomato and optional avocado.

# SPANISH "RICE"

*The cauliflower retains a ricelike shape and texture in this innovative dish.*

1 head cauliflower
2 ripe tomatoes, diced
1 ripe avocado, peeled, pitted, and mashed or diced
1 orange bell pepper, diced
4 green onions, finely chopped
¼ cup chopped fresh cilantro
¼ cup cold-pressed extra-virgin olive oil
2 tablespoons freshly squeezed lemon juice
1 jalapeño chile, minced (optional)
1 tablespoon paprika
1 teaspoon chili powder
1 teaspoon sea salt

Grate the cauliflower in a food processor and transfer it to a large bowl. Add the tomatoes, avocado, bell pepper, green onions, cilantro, olive oil, lemon juice, optional chile, paprika, chili powder, and sea salt to taste. Mix well.

# "SAUTÉED" MUSHROOMS

YIELD: 1 SERVING

*Nama Shoyu is raw, unpasteurized Japanese soy sauce. Look for it in natural food stores or online.*

1 portobello mushroom
Nama Shoyu

Remove and discard the stem of the mushroom and clean the cap. Slice the cap into squares or strips. Sprinkle with Nama Shoyu to taste and let marinate for 2 hours before serving.

# CHINESE BROCCOLI WITH PINE NUTS

**YIELD: 4 SERVINGS**

*Habanero chiles, which are closely related to Scotch bonnet chiles, are among the hottest chiles on the planet. Use them with care!*

3 cups chopped broccoli florets
$\frac{1}{2}$ cup pine nuts
1 ripe avocado, peeled and pitted
$\frac{1}{4}$ cup cold-pressed extra-virgin olive oil
1 tablespoon freshly squeezed lemon juice
1 habanero chile
1 clove garlic
$\frac{1}{2}$ teaspoon sea salt

Combine the broccoli and $\frac{1}{4}$ cup of the pine nuts in a large bowl. Place the remaining $\frac{1}{4}$ cup of pine nuts and the avocado, olive oil, lemon juice, chile, and garlic in a blender or food processor and process until smooth. Pour over the broccoli mixture and season with sea salt to taste. Marinate for 45 minutes in the refrigerator before serving.

# MARINATED VEGGIES

**YIELD: 1 SERVING**

*This fresh-tasting salad really hits the spot in hot weather.*

1 medium-size yellow summer squash, chopped
1 medium-size zucchini, chopped
Juice of 2 lemons

Place the squash and zucchini in a large bowl and sprinkle them with the lemon juice. Marinate for 4 to 6 hours before serving.

# Cauliflower "Mashed Potatoes"

**YIELD: 5 SERVINGS**

*Cauliflower tastes amazingly like potatoes in this recipe. The thyme and lemon give this dish a savory yet fresh taste.*

3 cups cauliflower florets
1/2 cup pine nuts
1/2 cup fresh thyme leaves
1/4 cup freshly squeezed lemon juice
2 cloves garlic
Sea salt
Olive oil

Combine all of the ingredients in a food processor, adding salt and olive oil to taste. Process until the mixture is the consistency of mashed potatoes. Add a small amount of water, if necessary, to facilitate processing and achieve the desired consistency.

# Mushroom Gravy

**YIELD: 8 TO 12 SERVINGS**

*Serve this over Cauliflower "Mashed Potatoes" (above).*

4 portobello mushrooms
1 jar (8 ounces) raw almond butter
1 cup water
2 ripe plum tomatoes, coarsely chopped
1 medium-size red onion, coarsely chopped
2 cloves garlic, coarsely chopped
Sea salt

Remove and discard the stems of the mushroom. Clean and coarsely chop the caps. Transfer to a food process along with all of the remaining ingredients, adding salt to taste. Process until completely smooth.

# PINE NUT PUDDING

*Dates are the perfect base for raw puddings and desserts. Use them whenever you need something sweet to hold other ingredients together.*

1 cup pine nuts
1 cup pitted soft dates
1 cup water
Ground nutmeg (optional)

Place the pine nuts, dates, and water in a blender and process until completely smooth. Sprinkle with nutmeg, if desired.

# APPLESAUCE

*Banana in applesauce? You'll love it.*

3 apples, cored and coarsely chopped
1 ripe banana, cut into 4 or 5 large pieces
4 pitted soft dates
$1/4$ cup water
Ground nutmeg (optional)

Place the apples, banana, dates, and water in a blender and process until completely smooth. Sprinkle with nutmeg, if desired.

# Paul's Coconut Fruit Pie

*I've perfected this pie recipe over the years, and it's a hit with my friends and family.*

CRUST:

> 2 cups chopped walnuts
>
> 2 cups chopped pecans
>
> 1/2 cup freshly squeezed orange juice
>
> 7 pitted medjool dates
>
> 1 ripe banana, thinly sliced
>
> 1 ripe mango, peeled, pitted, and thinly sliced

FILLING:

> 3 1/2 cups young coconut meat (about 4 young coconuts)
>
> 1 cup young coconut juice (from about 1 young coconut)
>
> 1 ripe banana (optional)
>
> 6 pitted medjool dates
>
> 1 tablespoon psyllium powder
>
> Shredded coconut and raisins or pine nuts

To prepare the crust, place the walnuts, pecans, orange juice, and dates in a food processor and process until the mixture has the consistency of pastry dough. Press the mixture into an 8-inch glass pie plate to form the crust. Arrange the banana and mango slices over the bottom of the crust.

To prepare the filling, place the coconut meat, coconut juice, optional banana, dates, and psyllium powder in a blender and process until completely smooth. Pour into the pie crust. Garnish the edges of the pie with shredded coconut and raisins or pine nuts.

# BLUEBERRY PIE

*Psyllium powder is derived from the herb Plantago psyllium. It adds fiber to foods and has been shown to lower cholesterol levels.*

CRUST:

- 2 cups pecans
- 2 cups walnuts
- 1 cup pitted dates
- $1/4$ teaspoon freshly squeezed orange juice
- 1 ripe banana, thinly sliced

FILLING:

- 4 cups blueberries
- 3 ripe bananas, cut into 4 or 5 pieces
- 1 cup pitted dates
- 1 cup cashews
- 1 tablespoon psyllium powder
- Shredded coconut

To prepare the crust, place the pecans, walnuts, dates, and orange juice in a food processor and process until the mixture has the consistency of pastry dough. Press the mixture into an 8-inch glass pie plate to form the crust. Arrange the banana slices over the bottom of the crust and set aside.

To prepare the filling, place the blueberries, bananas, dates, cashews, and psyllium powder in a blender and process until smooth. Pour over the banana slices in the crust. Decorate the pie with shredded coconut.

# Strawberry "Cheesecake"

**YIELD: 8 SERVINGS**

*Yes, you can even enjoy cheesecake on a raw diet.*

CRUST:

  2 cups pecans or walnuts

  1 cup pitted dates, soaked in water for 5 minutes and drained

  1/4 cup ground flaxseeds

  1/4 teaspoon sea salt

  1/4 teaspoon vanilla extract

FILLING:

  3 cups cashews, soaked in water for at least 1 hour and drained

  3/4 cup raw agave syrup

  1/2 cup freshly squeezed lemon juice

  1/4 cup raw coconut butter (optional)

  1 teaspoon vanilla extract

  1/2 teaspoon sea salt

TOPPING:

  2 cups frozen strawberries

  1 cup pitted dates, soaked in water for 10 minutes and drained

  1/4 cup almond milk (see Nut Milk, page 121)

To prepare the crust, place the pecans in a food processor and process or pulse until finely chopped. Add the dates, flaxseeds, salt, and vanilla extract and process until the mixture forms a ball. Turn out into an 8-inch springform pan and press the mixture into a crust.

To prepare the filling, place the cashews, agave syrup, lemon juice, optional coconut butter, vanilla extract, and sea salt in a food processor. Process until completely smooth, adding 1 teaspoon of water at a time, if necessary, to thin the mixture and obtain the desired consistency. Pour into the crust. Tap the pan on the counter to remove any air bubbles.

To prepare the topping, place the strawberries, dates, and almond milk in a food processor and process until very smooth. Pour over the filling.

Freeze the cheesecake for several hours or until firm. To serve, remove the cheesecake from the springform pan while still frozen.

# DATE BALLS

**YIELD: 1 SERVING (3 DATE BALLS)**

*This is a nice little dessert recipe for one.*

  6 pitted medjool dates
  2 tablespoons unsweetened raw carob powder
  3 pecan halves
  Shredded coconut or sesame seeds

Place the dates and carob powder in a food processor and process until smooth. Form the mixture into balls. Place a pecan half in each ball, and roll the balls in shredded coconut or sesame seeds.

# MACADAMIA PUDDING

**YIELD: 2 CUPS**

*This sweet and luscious pudding is so simple—just nuts and dates. How could it not be delicious?*

  1 cup macadamia nuts
  1 cup pitted medjool dates
  1 cup water

Place all of the ingredients in a blender or food processor and process until smooth.

# RAW FUDGE

**YIELD: 10 TO 12 SERVINGS**

*If you've never eaten carob before, you'll be surprised at how the taste resembles cocoa. Agave syrup is a by-product of the production of mescal, a liquor distilled from the agave plant. The syrup is sold in natural food stories. Be sure to get the raw syrup, not the pasteurized version.*

FUDGE:

    6 medium-size ripe avocados

    2 cups raw agave syrup

    1$\frac{1}{2}$ cups unsweetened raw carob powder

    1$\frac{1}{2}$ cups cold water

    2 teaspoons vanilla extract

TOPPINGS:

    Strawberries and/or ripe bananas

    Mint leaves

    Sprinkle of ground cinnamon

Combine all of the fudge ingredients in a food processor and process until smooth and thick, with a consistency like pudding. Serve with your choice of toppings.


# BANANA "ICE CREAM"

**YIELD: 1 SERVING**

*I'd be hard-pressed to find a more delicious dessert that is this simple to make.*

    2 ripe bananas, frozen

Place the frozen bananas in a blender or food processor. Process until smooth, adding a small amount of water, if necessary, to achieve the desired consistency.

# Banana Drink

*This tastes like you're drinking a dessert.*

   1 ripe banana, cut into 2 or 3 pieces
   2 pitted dates
   1/2 cup water

Place all of the ingredients in a blender and process until smooth.


# Coconut Shake

YIELD: 2 TO 3 SERVINGS

*Young coconuts have more meat, are more tender, and contain more water than older coconuts, so they're tastier and more nutritious. Look for them in Asian or Mexican markets or order them online.*

   Meat from 3 young coconuts
   Water from 1 young coconut (about 1 cup)

Place the coconut meat in a blender or food processor. Add the coconut water and process until smooth.


# Coconut Avocado Drink

YIELD: 1 SERVING

*Coconut and avocado make a surprisingly good combination.*

   Meat and water from 1 young coconut
   1 ripe avocado, peeled and pitted

Place the coconut meat, coconut water, and avocado in a blender and process until smooth.

# COCONUT, SPINACH, AND AVOCADO DRINK

**YIELD: 2 CUPS**

*Spinach gives this unusual drink more depth of flavor.*

Meat and water from 1 young coconut
1 cup spinach leaves or other greens
1 ripe avocado, peeled and pitted

Place the coconut meat and water in a blender and process until smooth. Add the spinach and avocado and process until smooth.

# BLENDED MANGO DRINK

**YIELD: 1 SERVING**

*Another dessertlike drink with incredible freshness of flavor.*

2 very ripe mangoes, peeled and pitted
Raw tahini or raw cashew butter (optional)

Place the mangoes in a blender and process until smooth. If desired, add the optional tahini or cashew butter to taste (for a richer, creamier drink) and process again until well combined.

# BANANA TAHINI DRINK

**YIELD: 1 SERVING**

*Nutty-tasting tahini is a great addition to just about anything.*

1 ripe banana, cut into 4 or 5 pieces
1 cup water
2 tablespoons raw tahini

Place all of the ingredients in a blender and process until very smooth.

# Nut Milk

*Medjool dates are native to Morocco, but they are now also grown in the United States. They are considered the queen of dates because of their large size and extraordinary sweetness.*

$1/2$ cup soaked almonds or other nut of choice

1 cup water

4 pitted medjool dates

Place the almonds and water in blender. Add the dates and blend until smooth. Strain through cheesecloth and discard the residue.

# "Egg" Nog

*No, this is nothing like the egg nog you're used to—it's better.*

1 vanilla bean

2 cups almond milk (see Nut Milk, above)

1 cup macadamia nuts

1 ripe banana, cut into 4 or 5 pieces

$1/2$ cup raw honey

1 tablespoon ground cinnamon

1 teaspoon ground nutmeg

$1/4$ teaspoon turmeric

Slice the vanilla bean in half lengthwise with the tip of a sharp knife. Scrape the seeds from each half into a blender and discard the bean. Add all of the remaining ingredients to the blender and process until smooth.

# BLENDED SALAD

*For better digestion, try drinking your salads instead of chewing them. Here's one of my favorites.*

  1 cup spinach or lettuce leaves
  1 cup sunflower sprouts (optional)
  1 ripe avocado, peeled and pitted
  1 ripe tomato, coarsely chopped
  1/2 red bell pepper, cored, seeded, and cut into 4 or 5 pieces (optional)
  1/2 medium-size cucumber, cut into 3 or 4 pieces
  1 stalk celery, cut into 3 or 4 pieces
  Juice of 1/2 lemon
  1 teaspoon flaxseed oil or cold-pressed extra-virgin olive oil (optional)

Combine all of the ingredients in a food processor or blender and process until smooth.

# Resources

**Paul Nison**
P.O. Box 16156
West Palm Beach, FL 33416
561-337-9299
www.paulnison.com
E-mail: paul@rawlife.com

*This is the official website of author and raw food chef Paul Nison. It has many resources for Paul's teachings and his lecture schedule.*

**Raw Life, Inc.**
P.O. Box 16156
West Palm Beach, FL 33416
866-729-7285
www.rawlife.com
E-mail: paul@rawlife.com

*This is the best website for health books on all topics, including raw food diets and books to help improve your spiritual health. It also has a good selection of the highest-quality raw food health snacks, foods, and supplements.*

**Torah Life Ministries**
P.O. Box 16156
West Palm Beach, FL 33416
561-337-9299
www.torahlifeministries.org

*Torah Life Ministries, Inc. is a nonprofit ministry teaching the word of YHWH, proclaiming the Good News of Yeshua, and supporting the healing of all by revealing a more excellent way. It is our heart's desire to help fellow believers understand the important health message found in the Scriptures.*

**Hippocrates Health Institute**
1443 Palmdale Court
West Palm Beach, FL 33411
561-471-8876
www.hippocratesinst.com

*Mention that Paul Nison referred you and you will receive a 5 percent discount on the tuition fee for the program.*

**Health Research Books**
www.healthresearchbooks.com
888-844-2386

*This is the world's largest publisher of rare and unusual health-related books.*

# Other Books by Paul Nison

*The Raw Life: Becoming Natural in an Unnatural World*

*Raw Knowledge: Enhance the Powers of Your Mind, Body and Soul*

*Raw Knowledge Part 2: Interviews with Health Achievers*

*Healing Inflammatory Bowel Disease: The Cause and Cure of Crohn's Disease and Ulcerative Colitis*

*Health According to the Scriptures: Experience the Joy of Health According to Our Creator*

# Bibliography

Anderson, Richard. *Cleanse & Purify Thyself.* Mt. Shasta, CA: Christobe Publishing, 1988.

Balch, Phyllis and James. *Prescription for Nutritional Healing, 3rd edition,* New York, NY: Avery Publishing/Penguin Putman Inc., 2000.

Bogdonovich, Ruza. *The Cure is in the Cause.* Genoa, NV: Spirit Spring Foundation, Inc., 2001.

Boutenko, Victoria. *Green for Life.* Canada: Raw Family Publishing, 2005.

Bragg, Paul C. *The Miracle of Fasting.* Santa Barbara, CA: Health Science, 1966.

Campbell, T. Colin and Thomas M. Campbell II. *The China Study.* Dallas, TX: Benbella Books, 2006.

Carque, Otto. *Rational Diet.* Pomeroy, Washington: Health Research Books, 1923.

———. *Vital Facts About Foods.* Pomeroy Washington: Health Research Books, 1940.

Clement, Brian R., with Theresa Foy Digeronimo. *Living Foods for Optimum Health.* Rocklin, CA: Prima Publishing, 1996.

Cousens, Gabriel. *Conscious Eating.* Santa Rosa, CA: Vision Books International, 1992.

———. *Rainbow Green Live-Food Cuisine.* Santa Rosa, California: North Atlantic Books and Essene Vision Books, 2003.

Dewey, Edward Hookey. *No Breakfast Plan and The Fasting Cure.* Pomeroy, Washington: Health Research Books 1900.

Ehret, Arnold. *The Cause and Cure of Disease.* Dobbs Ferry, New York: Erhet Literature Publishing Company, 2001.

———. *The Mucusless Diet Healing System.* New York, New York: Benedict Lust Publications, 2002.

———. *Rational Fasting.* New York: Benedict Lust Publications, 2002.

Estes, St. Louis. *Raw Food and Health.* Pomeroy, Washington: Health Research Books, 1923.

Hotema, Hilton. *How I Lived to be Ninety.* Pomeroy, Washington: 1966.

———. *Live Better.* Pomeroy, Washington: Health Research Books, 1963.

———. *Live Longer.* Pomeroy, Washington: Health Research Books, 1959.

———. *Long Life in Florida.* Pomeroy, Washington: Health Research Books, 1962.

———. *Man's Higher Consciousness.* Pomeroy, Washington: Health Research Books, 1962.

———. *Why Do We Age?* Pomeroy, Washington: Health Research Books, 1959.

Howell, Edward. *Enzyme Nutrition.* Wayne, NJ: Avery Publication, 1985.

———. *Food Enzymes for Health & Longevity (2nd Edition).* Twin Lakes, Wisconsin: Lotus Press, 1994.

Just, Adolf. *Return To Nature.* Pomeroy, Washington: Health Research Books, 1903.

Kordich, Jay. *Juiceman's Power of Juicing.* New York, New York: Warner Books, 1993.

Kulvinskas, Viktoras. *Survival Into the 21st Century*. Fairfield, Iowa: 21st Century Publications, 1975.

Lyman, Howard. *Mad Cowboy*. New York: Scribner, 1998.

Meyerowitz, Steve. *Food Combining and Digestion*. Great Barrington, Massachusetts: Sprout House, 2002.

Moritz, Andreas. *The Amazing Liver & Gallbladder Flush*. Landrum, South Carolina: Ener-chi.com, 2005.

Nungesser.Charles, Coralanne and George Nungesser. *How We All went Raw*. In the Beginning Health Ministry, Mesa Arizona.

Pearson, R. B. *Fasting and Man's Correct Diet*. Pomeroy, Washington: Health Research Books, 1921.

Pottenger, Francis M., Jr. *Pottenger's Cats*. La Mesa, CA: Price-Pottenger Nutrition Foundation, 1983.

Price, Weston A. *Nutrition & Physical Degeneration*. Santa Monica, CA: The Price-Pottenger Foundation, 1945/1972.

Richter, John T. & Vera M. Richter. *Nature the Healer*. Pomeroy, Washington: Spirit Spring Foundation, Inc., 1936.

Robbins, John. *Diet for a New America*. Walpole, New Hampshire: Stillpoint Publishing, 1987.

Rocine, Victor G. *Eating for Beauty*. Pomeroy, Washington: Health Research Books, 1929.

Romano, Rita. *Dining in the Raw*. New York, New York: Kensington Books, 1992.

Santillo, Humbart. *Food Enzymes, The Missing Link to Radiant Health*. Prescott, Arizona: Hohm Press, 1987.

Schaeffer, Severen L. *Instinctive Nutrition*. Berkeley, California: Celestial Arts, 1987.

Shelton, Herbert. *Fasting Can Save your Life*. Tampa, Florida: Natural Hygiene Press, 1964.

———. *Food Combining Made Easy*. San Antonio, Texas: Willow Publishing, 1982.

Soria, Cherie. *Angel Food*. Santa Barbara, California: Hearstar Productions, 1996.

Tilden, J. H. *Toxemia Explained*. Pomeroy, Washington: Health Research Books, 1997.

Walker, N. W. *Become Younger*. Phoenix, AZ: Norwalk Press, 1949.

———. *Fresh Vegetable and Fruit Juices*. Phoenix, AZ: O'Sullivan Woodside and Co., 1978.

Wigmore, Ann. *Be Your Own Doctor*. Wayne, NJ: Avery Pub. Group, 1982.

———. *The Blending Book*. New York, New York: Avery Publishing, 1997.

———. *The Hippocrates Diet*. Wayne, NJ: Avery Pub. Group, 1984.

Young, Robert O. *The pH Miracle*. New York, New York: Warner Book, 2002.

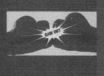 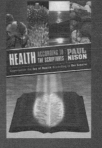
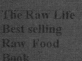 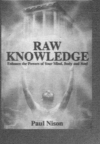

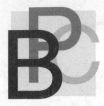
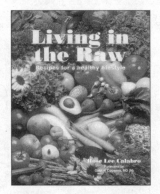
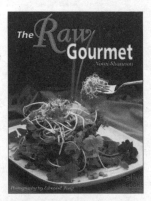
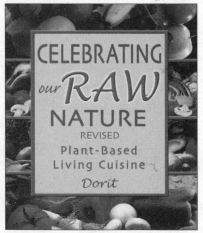
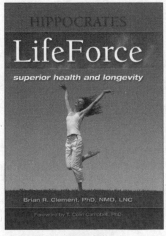